Jane Rossiter graduated with a BSc Hons in Home Economics from the University of Surrey in 1976. She spent two years in consumer market research and a further four years as Health Education Officer with a North London Area Health Authority, promoting healthy eating for kids.

Since 1984 she has taught Home Economics at adult classes on the themes of 'eating for health' and 'wholefood cookery'. Jane teaches Home Economics at a secondary girls school teaching pupils between the age of eleven and eighteen. She is married with two children.

Rosemary Seddon qualified as a State Registered Dietitian in 1973 and then worked in therapeutic dietetics at Northwick Park Hospital, Harrow, Middlesex where her responsibilities included the Diabetic Clinic. Later she took up the post of Community Dietitian for the Harrow Health Authority and was involved in promoting good nutrition for children of all ages (in family clinics, GP surgeries, with health visitors and in schools).

Rosemary now works freelance, writing and lecturing on healthy eating and dietetics, and co-ordinating courses on treatment of obesity for a Health Authority. She has appeared on BBC TV's *Medical Express* programme. She is married with three children.

OPTIMA

THE DIABETIC KIDS' COOKBOOK

Jane Rossiter
and
Rosemary Seddon, SRD

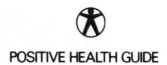

POSITIVE HEALTH GUIDE

To David, Rebecca, Thomas, Caroline and Alexander

First published in 1987 by Optima
Reprinted in 1992

Little, Brown and Company (UK) Limited
165 Great Dover Street
London
SE1 4YA

Designed and computer generated in Times by
The Design & Illustration Partnership

Printed by Toppan Printing Company (S) Pte Ltd, Singapore

CONTENTS

INTRODUCTION

Encouraging any child to enjoy a healthy diet is a challenging task, even more so if your child has diabetes.

You may be the parent of a newly diagnosed diabetic or an 'old hand' coming to grips with the new high-fibre, low-fat recommendations. This book aims to give you plenty of practical ideas on how the new healthy guidelines on diabetic diets can be incorporated in everyday meals, particularly in dishes that are popular with children.

This is not intended to be a do-it-yourself diabetic diet manual. Every child is unique and the advice of your own doctor, dietitian, nurse and the rest of the diabetic team is essential to help you to work out the best approach for your family. There is a lot to learn so do not expect to be an expert at once.

Begin by making sure you understand what diabetes is and how food and insulin are linked. This is the first and very important step in learning how to apply these guidelines to feeding your child.

Understanding diabetes

A clear understanding of diabetes is the key to its successful management in everyday life. By learning about the relationship between diet and insulin, and their effect on blood sugar levels, it is easier to achieve good control. This is essential for your child's health, both now and in the future.

Diabetes affects around 30,000 children in the UK. You may be surprised to hear that there are approximately 1,500 new diabetics under sixteen years old diagnosed each year, and all of these require treatment by insulin injection. It is encouraging to realize you are not the only parent facing the task of bringing up a diabetic child!

Diabetes mellitus, the correct term for the condition, is caused by a lack of insulin. This hormone is produced by the pancreas, a gland situated just below the stomach. Insulin is essential in the process of using sugar for energy. Sugary and starchy foods are digested mostly to glucose (a simple form of sugar) and absorbed into the bloodstream. The glucose is then converted to energy for all the body's activities. Apart from exercise, energy is also needed for breathing, heartbeat, warmth, digestion and brain function. Excess energy is converted to fat for storage.

When insulin is lacking, the body cannot obtain energy from the glucose in the blood. As a result the blood glucose level rises and glucose overflows into the urine. The body attempts to replace the fluid lost by causing the child to become thirsty, drink more and consequently make frequent trips to the toilet. If the thirst is quenched by sweet drinks, the condition is aggravated by increasing blood glucose levels further. Hunger and weight loss are a result of the body's inability to use the glucose for energy. Fat stores are broken down to provide some energy causing an excess of ketones (fat breakdown products) in the blood and urine. (The presence of ketones can be recognized by their distinctive smell of pear-drops.) Other symptoms may occur including repeated infections and feeling generally unwell. If the diabetes is not treated the child would become severely ill and eventually unconscious. Diabetes is diagnosed by testing the urine and blood levels of glucose (and ketones).

As yet there is no cure for diabetes; the treatment is to give insulin one or more times a day. This hormone would be digested if taken by mouth so it has to be given by injection. When a sugary or starchy food is eaten, the correct quantity of insulin to match this food would normally be released by the pancreas. If your child has diabetes, the right amount of insulin must be given to balance food eaten and energy used up in exercise each day. In the early weeks, a constant amount is decided for the daily insulin dose and the food eaten must match this. This is why diet is such an important part of the treatment of diabetes. It does not mean having to eat special foods or exactly the same foods every day; but it does involve controlling all foods containing sugar or starch, known as carbohydrates. Initially your child will find it easier to keep the amounts of insulin, food and exercise the same from one day to the next. But when you and your child are more practised at diabetes care, the insulin, food and exercise can be varied to suit day-to-day variations in lifestyle.

The diabetes that develops in childhood is known as juvenile onset diabetes, also called insulin dependent diabetes mellitus. This differs from the condition known as maturity onset diabetes which usually occurs in middle age but can rarely occur in older children. In this adult condition the pancreas produces insulin but it is ineffective. Treatment can usually be provided by diet alone or by tablets but these remedies will not help someone with juvenile onset diabetes.

Controlling the carbohydrates is the most essential aspect of dietary treatment but it is only part of the story in giving your child a healthy diet. A child needs the right foods for normal growth (such as those containing protein, vitamins and minerals). Overweight should be avoided. In addition, recent guidelines for diabetics have recommended a healthier diet with more fibre and less fat.

Applying all these considerations in daily life – at meal-times and for snacks, either at home or at school, for parties or on holiday – may seem daunting at first. The following sections give practical advice to help you with this challenging task.

A healthy diet for diabetic kids

Controlling the carbohydrates
The word carbohydrate is used to describe sugary and starchy foods. Many foods contain carbohydrate – from obvious ones like sugar, sweets, bread and biscuits to less obvious foods like fruit and milk (see Table 1, page 10).

When sugar and starch are eaten, both are broken down by digestion to simple sugars, mostly in the form of glucose. This is because starch is made up of chains of glucose molecules and most sugars are made up of two molecules, one of which is glucose. After digestion glucose is absorbed into the blood and eventually used for energy, with the help of insulin.

The carbohydrate your child eats each day must be balanced by a correct dose of insulin and your child must continue to eat the same amount of carbohydrate daily to match the insulin dose unless the dose is altered. All carbohydrates end up mainly as glucose in the body so it is not necessary to eat the same foods each day, just foods with the equivalent amount of carbohydrate.

This does not mean you have to get out a calculator or book of food tables before preparing your child's meals! A universal system of carbohydrate exchanges has been devised which most diabetics use. Foods are calculated in portions containing 10 grams (g) of carbohydrate. One portion or exchange can simply be swapped for another. Using this system for your child's diet is explained on page 12.

Well-controlled diabetes means the blood glucose levels are kept as near as possible to within normal range (4–7 mmol/litre). This can be achieved by a correct balance of insulin and diet and checked by regular blood and urine tests. Consistently raised blood sugar or a dramatic swing shows the diabetes is not under control and is a recipe for poor health.

Some carbohydrates are better for diabetic control than others. The more slowly that glucose is absorbed into the bloodstream, the better. In the table overleaf the carbohydrate foods are divided into three 'traffic light' sections depending on their effect on the absorption rate of glucose.

High-fibre starchy carbohydrates, shown in the green section, are best. Fibre is not digested and it acts like a sponge slowing down the absorption rate of glucose. Foods with a high-fibre content include wholemeal bread and flour, whole grain breakfast cereals, brown rice, wholemeal pasta, fruit and most vegetables, particularly pulses like dried beans, peas and lentils. The fibre in cooked dried beans and pulses (such as haricot, red kidney, lentils and chick peas) seems to control diabetes even better than cereal or vegetable fibre. Apart from canned baked beans, pulses do not feature frequently in many children's diets. Look for new ways of incorporating them into your child's meals – the recipe section gives you lots of ideas!

The amber section shows carbohydrates which are lower in fibre like white bread and flour, and refined breakfast cereals. Although they do not have such a slow absorption rate as high-fibre foods, these starchy foods are preferable to sugar and sugary foods because they are absorbed more slowly into the bloodstream. In fact they can certainly have a place in your child's diet provided you also include high-fibre foods.

The red section includes all foods containing sugar, such as sweetened drinks, sweets, chocolate, cakes, jam, marmalade and honey. Sugar and sugary foods are absorbed very quickly by the body and therefore give very poor diabetic control. These foods should normally be avoided in your child's diet, although there are times when they can be eaten, for example, before exercise (see page 25), on special occasions (see page 32), and during illness (see page 27). A small amount of sugar in baking recipes may be allowed provided it is taken with foods high in fibre (see page 34).

Children usually adapt much more quickly than newly diagnosed adults to the removal of sugar as a sweetener, for example, in tea or on breakfast cereals. There are special diabetic products made without sugar to help soften the blow of avoiding these foods. As well as sugar-free sweeteners, there are diabetic squashes, drinks, sweets and preserves. These are discussed in greater detail on page 33.

Diabetes is managed by controlling the carbohydrates, not restricting them. The original treatment for diabetes reduced carbohydrates to unreasonably low levels. This was not only impractical but also unhealthy as diabetics often turned to high-fat foods to make up their energy needs.

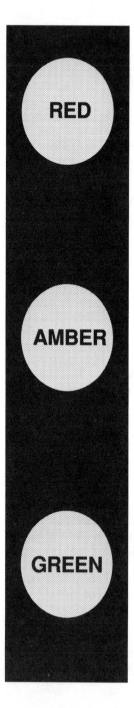

Carbohydrate foods

Sugary foods

White and brown sugar, sweets, chocolates, toffees, peppermints

Fruit squash, fizzy drinks, cola

Jam, marmalade, honey, lemon curd, syrup, treacle

Sugar-coated breakfast cereals, canned fruit in syrup

Cakes, sweet biscuits, instant desserts, mousse, jelly, condensed milk, fancy ice cream

Low-fibre starchy foods

White bread and flour, white rice, white pasta

Cornflakes, Rice Krispies, Special K

Cornflour, arrowroot, pudding rice, semolina

Plain biscuits, cream crackers

Fruit juice

Potatoes, chips, crisps

High-fibre foods

Wholemeal bread and flour

Weetabix, Shredded Wheat, Puffed Wheat, All Bran, Bran Flakes, Shreddies, porridge oats, unsweetened muesli

Potatoes, jacket or eaten with skin

Brown rice, wholemeal pasta (spaghetti, lasagne etc)

Wholemeal or bran crispbreads and biscuits

Oatcakes, digestive biscuits

Vegetables especially cooked dried beans

Fresh fruit, canned fruit in natural juice or water

Dried fruit

Remember the important thing is to balance the injected insulin, which is absorbed slowly into the blood throughout the day, with regular meals and snacks containing a constant amount of carbohydrate. Your own child's daily carbohydrate needs should have been individually worked out by your dietitian and doctor in discussion with you. The aim is that your child should be eating roughly the same amount of carbohydrate as he did before (though this depends on hunger prior to diagnosis). The difference will be in the type of carbohydrate: minimal sugar, less refined starchy foods and more fibre-rich ones. In fact he may find the new diet so satisfying he has difficulty in eating the required amount! Newly diagnosed diabetics are often ravenously hungry but their appetite usually settles down after the first few weeks.

Foods with a high-fibre content are not only best for diabetics. Fibre has a beneficial effect on digestion by increasing the rate of food passing through the intestine, thus preventing constipation and other disorders of the bowel. Current nutritional recommendations advise us all to increase the fibre in our diet and to reduce the sugar intake. You will do the whole family a favour in long-term health by changing to high-fibre foods and cutting down on sugar and sugary foods. This will also minimize the contrast between your diabetic child's meals and the rest of the family.

How much carbohydrate?
Your child's daily carbohydrate allowance depends on many factors: age, sex, height, weight, activity and normal appetite. This is why your dietitian will have assessed quite carefully what he had been eating at home. The idea of providing a generous carbohydrate intake with the emphasis on high-fibre foods is fairly recent. In fact, if you are the parent of a child who has been diabetic for some time, you may have noticed an increase in his carbohydrate allowance.

A diet with a higher proportion of carbohydrate, mostly from high-fibre foods and more pulses, has been shown to give better diabetic control. It also prevents the fat intake from being too high because more of the energy needs are being met by carbohydrate. Current recommendations for diabetics suggest at least half of the total energy intake (or calories) should come from carbohydrate. Achieving this figure in an adult diet has been clearly explained in another book in the Positive Health Guide series – *The Diabetics' Diet Book*. For children, however, reaching this high quantity of carbohydrate is more difficult. The sheer bulk may be just too much for a child's appetite. In practice, dietitians are finding that for a diabetic child it is best to emphasize the need to eat the right type and quantity of carbohydrate, while encouraging high-fibre foods where possible. As the child grows older, the teenage appetite may be able to manage a greater proportion of carbohydrate in the diet. (This is in addition to the increased quantity which is adjusted with age).

The day's carbohydrate must be evenly distributed to coincide with the insulin being slowly absorbed from the injection site. It is usually divided between the three main meals (breakfast, lunch and evening meal) with smaller amounts at three snacks (midmorning, afternoon and bedtime).

If insulin is given by two injections a day, then the breakfast and evening meal may be larger. It is important that breakfast is taken shortly after the morning injection and an adequate bedtime snack (including high-fibre carbohydrate for slower absorption) is essential to cover the night-time needs. The other meals and snacks should be at a similar time each day. Because the insulin is working all the time it is not wise to have long gaps between meals without a snack as this could cause blood glucose levels to go too low. This is called hypoglycaemia (see page 24 for treatment). Some older children may be using the new insulin 'pen' which allows a greater flexibility in the timing of meals and it means that snacks may not be necessary. But a meal must be taken within 30 minutes of using the 'pen' injection.

Checking blood glucose levels by regular blood or urine tests at different times of the day will show you if the insulin and carbohydrate are balanced. A slightly different distribution of carbohydrate may achieve better control. Remember that blood glucose levels are also affected by exercise, excitement, emotional stress and illness.

Counting the carbohydrate

The thought of balancing the different carbohydrate foods in your child's diet may make you feel like a juggler with too many clubs in the air at once! In fact, you will be surprised how quickly you will adjust to counting the carbohydrates. Your child may even get the hang of it quicker than you.

Each meal should consist of carbohydrate foods totalling the suggested amount on the day's distribution as well as foods that do not contain carbohydrate such as meat and vegetables. Adding up the carbohydrate values of foods is simplified by the system that uses lists of food portions containing 10 g carbohydrate (see page 117). A meal can therefore be made up of a number of portions and different foods can be swapped or exchanged, provided they have the same carbohydrate value. For example, a 25 g/¾ oz slice of bread could be exchanged for 1 apple or 1 small potato or 1 glass of milk as all of these contain 10 g carbohydrate.

For simplicity 10 g carbohydrate portions are usually shortened to:
1 (carbohydrate) exchange
1 (carbohydrate) unit
1 (carbohydrate) portion
1 C10 portion

It does not matter which term you use as they all mean the same. For consistency we use the word 'exchange' in this book.

Using the exchange system means that variety in the diet is much easier to achieve. For example, a weekday lunch of ham sandwiches and an apple could be replaced by a Sunday meal of roast chicken and vegetables, banana and yoghurt as follows:

	Exchange		Exchange
Ham and tomato sandwich with 2 x 50 g/1½ oz slices *wholemeal bread*	4	Chicken, Brussels sprouts, 150 g/5 oz baked *potato*	3
1 *apple*	1	1 *banana*	1
		1 natural *yoghurt*	1
	5		5

(Foods containing carbohydrate are in italics.)

A bedtime snack of 2 exchanges could consist of:

	Exchange		Exchange
1 apple	1	1 x 50 g/1½ oz slice wholemeal bread (as Marmite sandwich)	2
1 digestive biscuit	1		
	2		
			2
1 Weetabix	1		
200 ml/7 fl oz milk	1		
	2		

Although it is not necessary to eat the same foods at each meal but just the same amount of carbohydrate, in practice your child probably eats some foods consistently each day – for example, the same amounts of cereal and toast at breakfast or a regular sandwich meal.

Table 2 (see overleaf) shows sample menus of a day's diet and carbohydrate distribution for two children of different ages. Remember these are only average figures and not intended to replace the guidelines given by your own dietitian and doctor to suit your child's individual needs.

When you are first using the exchange list, always weigh the food on accurate scales. Lightweight portable diet scales are available for weighing small portions of food. It is strongly recommended that you use metric measures, that is grams (g) and millilitres (ml). Imperial measures (ounces – oz and fluid ounces – fl oz) when calculated from the metric are often in fractions of an ounce and are less easy to measure accurately. 1 oz = 28.35 g, or for a rough conversion 25 g or 30 g, and in the recipes we have used 30 g. Some foods can be measured with reasonable accuracy using standard measuring spoons (a set of four is available from the British Diabetic Association, see page 123). Ordinary household tablespoons and teaspoons vary tremendously.

Gradually you will learn to judge amounts of frequently used foods such as bread, potatoes or breakfast cereal, without having to weigh these every time. You may even find a particular cup that measures out 2 exchanges of a favourite cereal. It is a good idea to check your 'judgements' on the scales from time to time. For example, 1 slice of bread can vary between 1 and 2 exchanges.

Let your child learn the basic foods by heart too and encourage him to weigh and judge the exchanges himself. It is quite fun to guess the weight of a particular food especially if his estimation is nearer than Mum's. It is important that your child becomes confident in estimating portions, especially when eating away from home. Learning to take responsibility in managing the diet is important as a child grows older.

Get into the habit of using a simplified term like 'exchanges' rather than 10 g carbohydrate. It is possible to get confused between the weight of food in grams and the carbohydrate value in grams. Which looks easier to you?

	Measure	Carbohydrate
Wholemeal bread	25 g	10 g
Wholemeal bread	1 small, thin slice	1 exchange

Sample menu plans (Remember these are only examples; your child has individual needs)
1 sample school day's meals for a five-year-old girl having 180 g carbohydrate (18 exchanges) 1700 kcal/7010 kJ, 80 g protein, 80 g fat, 25 g fibre

Day's milk allowance for drinks and cereal	Exchanges
400 ml/14 fl oz whole milk	2

Breakfast

Shredded Wheat (30 g/1 oz) with milk from allowance	1
1 glass (100 ml/3½ fl oz) orange juice	1
1 x 25 g/¾ oz slice wholemeal bread with	
polyunsaturated margarine and Marmite	2
	4

Mid-morning (at playtime)

1 apple	1

Packed lunch

1 wholemeal bap spread with margarine and	
Smoked mackerel pâté (see page 77)	2
1 small carton natural yoghurt	1
Crisps (15 g/½ oz)	1
Water or can of sugar-free drink	—
	4

Mid-afternoon

Sugar-free squash	
1 Apricot oatcake (see page 98)	1

Evening meal

Jacket potato (100 g/3½ oz) with small knob butter	2
1 Chicken burger (see page 51)	1
Green beans, carrots	
Banana ice cream (see page 88)	1
Tea, water or sugar-free squash	—
	4

Bedtime

Remainder of milk from allowance with 2 tsp Ovaltine	1
1 digestive biscuit	1
	2
	18

Sample menu plans
Sample non–school day's meals for a ten-year-old boy having 250 g
carbohydrate (25 exchanges) 2050 kcal/8460 kJ, 100 g protein, 75 g fat,
45 g fibre

Day's milk allowance for drinks and cereal	Exchanges
600 ml/1 pint semi-skimmed milk	3

Breakfast

2 Weetabix with milk from allowance	2
1 glass grapefruit juice (120 ml/4 fl oz)	1
1 x 50 g/1½ oz slice wholemeal bread as toast with	
polyunsaturated margarine and diabetic marmalade	2
Tea with milk from allowance	—
	5

Mid-morning

2 digestive biscuits	2

Lunch

Spaghetti bolognese (see page 55)	4
Green salad	
Fresh pear	1
Water or sugar-free drink	—
	5

Mid-afternoon

Sugar-free drink	
Peanuts (30 g/1 oz) and raisins (30 g/1 oz)	2

Evening meal

Hearty bean soup (see page 42)	2
1 boiled egg	
1 x 50 g/1½ oz sliced wholemeal bread as toast	
with polyunsaturated margarine	2
1 slice Apple cake (see page 96)	1
Water or tea to drink	—
	5

Bedtime

1⅓ Shredded wheat with remainder of milk	2
1 banana	1
	—
	3
	25

All the recipes in this book are in multiples of 10 g carbohydrate exchanges or half divisions so that they can be easily fitted into your child's diet.

Additional carbohydrate exchange lists are available from the British Diabetic Association which also produces a comprehensive booklet on carbohydrate values of foods and drinks called *Countdown*. When you feel proficient at controlling the diet, this booklet will be useful in giving greater variety in your child's diet. Be wary of obtaining it too soon: the carbohydrate values are not expressed in multiples of 10 g and this can be very confusing when you are just starting out.

Growing up with healthy food

Getting the carbohydrate balance sorted out in your child's diet is your first priority but, of course, not all foods contain carbohydrate. Your child needs the right balance of other foods to keep healthy, grow normally, avoid being overweight and minimize the risk of heart disease in later life.

Food is made up of various nutrients, all of which have an essential role to play:

protein, vitamins and minerals – for growth and health;

carbohydrates, fats, and protein – for energy;

fibre – for the healthy working of the digestive system.

Carbohydrates, fats and protein are all used for energy so any of these taken in excess of your child's needs could lead to overweight. Energy is measured in kilocalories (or kiloJoules, the metric equivalent) so excess energy intake means excess calories. (For convenience, calories are calculated in units of 1,000, hence kilocalories.) To encourage you, the diets of diabetics are generally more healthy than those of other people because of their avoidance of sweets, sweetened drinks and other carbohydrate foods of poor nutritional value, and their emphasis on foods like bread (which, in addition to carbohydrate, provides B vitamins, iron, calcium, protein and fibre).

However, you should take care that your child's intake of fat is not too high. The high proportion of fat in our western diet is linked to an increased risk of coronary heart disease. Recent nutritional recommendations advise a lower fat intake for everyone, but this is especially important for diabetics who have a greater tendency to these problems. Previous diabetic diets which reduced carbohydrate intakes meant that diabetics were forced to turn to fat and protein foods to meet their energy (or calorie) need. It was quite common to recommend a breakfast of fried eggs and bacon to accompany the one slice of bread allowed, double cream regularly for dessert, or a hunk of cheese as a nil-carbohydrate snack. A far cry from today's suggestions to cut down on fat!

With the more generous carbohydrate allowance in your child's diet there is no need for these extra foods. In fact, you should look for ways to limit his fat intake. This is important for two reasons: as well as reducing the risk of heart disease, it will prevent overweight. If more of your child's energy (or calorie) intake is contributed by carbohydrate, then too much fat could lead to weight problems. Energy (or calories), from whatever source, eaten in excess of the body's needs are stored as fat and cause overweight (see page 23).

Foods supplying fat in the diet include spreading fats; cooking fats for frying, baking, etc; snack foods like crisps, nuts and biscuits; cream and some of the protein foods (see page 18).

Reducing fatty foods

Fats are made up of saturated and unsaturated fats. Foods high in saturated fats are mainly from animal sources such as dairy produce and the fat in meat. It is saturated fats which are linked to a greater risk of heart disease because they may cause a rise in blood cholesterol levels in some individuals. Unsaturated fats, of which there are two types (mono- and poly-), do not have this effect. In fact, polyunsaturated fats may actually cause a drop in raised blood levels of cholesterol. Vegetable oils, nuts and fish oils have a high content of unsaturated fats. It has not yet been proved that polyunsaturated fats benefit those with normal cholesterol levels. It is therefore recommended to limit all types of fatty foods, putting particular emphasis on cutting saturated fat intake. Foods containing unsaturated fats can be substituted for saturated fats but should not be eaten to excess themselves.

Spreading fats Change from using butter every day to either a polyunsaturated margarine or a low-fat spread. Get into the habit of 'scraping' the margarine on the bread and avoid excessive amounts in cooking. Margarine (and butter) are important sources of vitamins A and D for your child so it would not be wise to cut them out altogether.

Polyunsaturated margarine has the same calorie content as butter and ordinary margarine but low-fat spread has half or less of their calorie value because it is partly composed of water.

Cooking fats Cut down your child's consumption of fried food as much as you can. Wherever possible use alternative methods of cooking such as grilling. Non-stick pans need a minimal amount of fat for frying. Instead of lard or dripping, change over to vegetable oils such as sunflower, corn, soya or safflower; avoid blended or mixed vegetable oil because both tend to be higher in saturated fats than pure vegetable oil. When roasting meat, wrap loosely in kitchen foil or brush lightly with oil. Re-use of vegetable oils for frying will gradually reduce their unsaturated fat content.

Most children love chips and it would be hard to banish this popular food completely from the diet (not forgetting to count the carbohydrate, of course). Chips are very high in fat so keep them for treats rather than every day. Ready-made 'oven' chips usually work out lower in fat than home-fried ones. It is much wiser to encourage a taste for baked potatoes (eat the skins as well for fibre), preferably without adding margarine (see page 73 for recipe ideas).

Fats also come from bakery products such as pastry, cakes, puddings and biscuits. Aim for fruit-based desserts rather than high-fat puddings. Where possible use polyunsaturated margarine in baking.

Cream, particularly double cream, has a low carbohydrate content so can be used without 'counting'. But like butter, it is rich in saturated fats, so keep it for special occasions.

Snacks Crisps and similar savoury snacks are high in fat. Nevertheless they are a popular and convenient sugar-free choice for between-meal snacks. The best

Carbohydrate-free foods

(Put emphasis on foods marked *. These are low in saturated fats.)

PROTEIN FOODS

These do not need to be measured but should be taken in moderate amounts similar to the servings for the rest of the family.

Meat
Chicken*, turkey*, duck
Beef, lamb, pork, ham*, bacon, veal
(Note: sausages, beefburgers, pâté and similar meat products usually contain carbohydrate)

Fish
White fish*, including cod, haddock, coley, plaice
Oily fish*, including mackerel, herring, sardine, tuna, pilchards, salmon
Shell fish*, including prawns, crab
(Note: fish fingers and fish cakes contain carbohydrate)

Eggs

Cheese
Hard cheese – Cheddar, Cheshire, Stilton
Moderate-fat cheese – Edam, Gouda, Brie, Camembert
Low-fat cheese – cottage cheese*, skimmed milk cheese (quark)*

Offal
Liver*, kidney*, sweetbreads*, tripe*, hearts*

FATTY FOODS

These should not be taken in excess:
Butter
Margarine: hard, soft and polyunsaturated*
Low-fat spread
Vegetable oil: sunflower*, soya*, corn*, safflower*
Lard, dripping
Cream (very low in carbohydrate)
Mayonnaise

compromise is to allow them not more than once a day (1-2 exchanges at maximum). A few brands of lower fat crisps are now available.

Fresh fruit, dried fruit and nuts, eg, peanuts, make good alternative snacks and also pre-dried cooked beans and peas (see page 113). Nuts are high in fat, though mostly of the unsaturated type, so allow them in moderation. Peanuts do not have a high carbohydrate content so a small handful need not be 'counted'. If eating more, eg, a packet, the carbohydrate content should be taken into account – 120 g/4^1/$_3$ oz for 1 exchange. (Nuts are not suitable for children under the age of three as they could choke on them. Discourage your child from dropping nuts into his mouth with his head tilted back for the same reason.)

How much protein food?

A child needs protein for the growth of every part of the body. Even when the body eventually stops growing, protein is needed for continuous renewal and repair of all tissues. Protein comes from both animal and vegetable sources. Foods from animal sources are meat, fish, eggs, milk, cheese, and yoghurt, whereas vegetable proteins are found in pulses (dried beans), nuts, bread and flour.

Protein foods also supply important vitamins and minerals in the diet. For example, milk and cheese are excellent sources of calcium, whereas meat, eggs and pulses provide iron. Animal protein foods contain a better quality protein than vegetable sources and they tend to be richer in other nutrients. But some of them have a high saturated fat content so should not be taken in excess. It is not necessary or advisable to avoid completely or reduce to dramatically low levels foods like meat, milk and eggs. They are nutritionally valuable in a child's diet but because of their fat content, it is wise to emphasize the leaner meats and lower-fat varieties of dairy produce.

Milk and milk products Milk contains carbohydrate in the form of lactose (a type of sugar) – 200 ml/7 fl oz is equivalent to 1 exchange (see page 119). Milk is an important source of protein and calcium, the mineral needed for making bones. For this reason, your child's carbohydrate allowance should include 400-600 ml/14 fl oz – 1 pint milk daily (2–3 exchanges) depending on age, and how much he likes it. Because of the high dairy fat content of milk and cheese, many lower-fat versions have been developed recently. For most children over the age of five, it is advisable to give semi-skimmed milk, which has a fat content halfway between ordinary pasteurized and skimmed milk. If you want to reduce the fat further, you could give skimmed milk but this is not advisable for most children, unless they are overweight. Skimmed milk is not recommended for children under the age of five; children in this age group would be advised to drink whole milk because they need the additional energy and vitamins.

Cheese is carbohydrate-free and an excellent source of calcium, but it does contain fat. Hard cheeses, like Cheddar, are the highest in fat, but their strong flavour means that less can be used in cooking. Medium-fat cheeses include Edam, Gouda, Brie and Camembert. Cottage cheese and skimmed milk cheese (often called quark) are low-fat cheeses. Lower-fat versions of Cheddar and Cheshire are also available. If your child enjoys the flavour of cheese, a small piece of mature Cheddar may be preferable to twice as much of a low-fat cheese. Grating cheese always makes it look more!

Like milk, yoghurt contains carbohydrate. Most small cartons of natural yoghurt are about 1 carbohydrate exchange. Choose yoghurts that are low in fat;

beware of the luxury versions which tend to have added cream. Adding fresh fruit or canned fruit in natural juice makes a popular dessert. The no–added–sugar, low-fat fruit yoghurts (eg, St Ivel 'Shape', Stapleton Farm, 'Diet Ski', 'Waistline') aimed at the slimmers' market have a carbohydrate value lower than 1 exchange for a small carton – that is, about 7 g carbohydrate depending on the brand. In comparison, 1 exchange of an ordinary fruit yoghurt is equivalent to one third to one half of a small carton. The carton usually states the carbohydrate value.

Although ice cream contains sugar, plain ice cream has a carbohydrate value of 1 exchange for 1 small brickette or scoop (50 g/1½ oz). It can make a pleasant change for dessert and is best used to accompany a high-fibre meal.

Meat Meat contains no carbohydrate but some meats are quite high in fat. The general rule is the leaner the meat, the better; cut off any visible fat and add the minimal amount in cooking. In many recipes the meat's own juices can be used for browning. Fat should be skimmed from stews and mince dishes.

Chicken, turkey and ham have less fat than most other meats so include them regularly. Lamb and pork tend to be higher in fat than lean beef. Liver and kidney are lower in fat and are rich in the mineral, iron.

Sausages, beefburgers, corned beef, luncheon meat, pâté and similar meat products are very high in fat. Do not serve more than once or twice a week. Grill sausages and beefburgers, and allow as much fat as possible to drain away. Low-fat versions of some of these products are now available.

Fish Fish is carbohydrate–free. White fish is very low in fat while oily fish contains mainly unsaturated fat. It is often neglected in children's diets, apart from fish fingers. Increase your family's consumption of fish, and let your child try the many varieties available.

Eggs It is the yolk in eggs that contains the saturated fat but eggs are an economical and highly nutritious food, free of carbohydrate. If your child enjoys eggs, 5–6 per week would not be excessive. Obviously this depends on other foods eaten and your child's appetite. If you are vegetarians, your child may eat more eggs instead of meat.

Pulses Dried beans, peas and lentils can be a meal alternative to meat as they also contain protein, iron and B vitamins. Their beneficial effect on carbohydrate control has already been mentioned. They do contain carbohydrate (see page 120) but with the more generous carbohydrate allowances, this should not mean missing out on something else. Experiment with recipes using pulses as the main ingredient and find out your child's favourites. If you have not used them much in your family's diet, set yourself a target of one main meal a week to begin with, more often when everyone gets used to the idea.

Make sure your child has one of these protein foods, in addition to the daily milk allowance, at two meals each day: Meat, fish, eggs, cheese, pulses. It is not essential to have a cooked breakfast. In fact a high-fibre cereal with milk followed by wholemeal bread or toast is probably a healthier choice for a diabetic child.

There is no need to feel that with the emphasis on avoiding excess meat, it would be better to be vegetarian. There is no necessity to give up meat completely. However, if you do wish your child to be vegetarian, it is perfectly possible for a diabetic to have an adequate diet, but I would advise that you allow milk, cheese and eggs.

Fruit and vegetables

Encourage your child to eat plenty of vegetables and fruit and to enjoy as great a variety as possible. Many are so low in carbohydrate that they may be eaten freely in the diet (see overleaf). Vegetables such as potatoes, parsnips, sweetcorn, dried peas and beans must be measured. An average portion of the majority of fruits contains around 10 g carbohydrate (1 exchange).

Vegetables and fruit are low in fat and calories and provide vitamins, minerals and fibre. Green vegetables, salad, potatoes, citrus and berry fruits are all important sources of vitamin C.

Many varieties of fruit are now available canned in water or natural juice and these make a handy and popular dessert. Dessert fruits (apples, pears, etc) make excellent between-meal snacks for diabetic children.

In contrast, fruit juices are not recommended to be taken between meals for diabetics. They contain very little fibre, so the fruit sugar is absorbed more quickly than from the whole fruit. It is wise to enjoy fruit juice as part of a meal, rather than a snack, because the absorption would be delayed. For drinks between meals give water and sugar-free squashes or fizzy drinks.

Miscellaneous free foods

The table overleaf also shows drinks, herbs, spices, sauces and so on which contain negligible carbohydrate and may be taken freely in the diet.

Salt – saint or sinner?

Another current recommendation on healthy eating is to cut down on salt. This is because high salt intakes have been linked with a greater risk of high blood pressure in some individuals. It would be wise to encourage your child, and indeed the whole family, to enjoy less salty food.

When cooking, add the minimum salt necessary for flavour, and discourage the use of the salt cellar at the table, especially if the food has already been prepared with salt. Convenience foods, smoked and preserved meats and fish, canned foods, cheese and sausages tend to be higher in salt (or other sodium compounds) than fresh or home-made equivalents. Aim to keep a reasonable balance in the diet, using fresh foods where possible. Crisps, nuts and other savoury snacks are also high in salt.

Many of these salty foods have already been mentioned because of their high fat content, so avoiding excess will give two nutritional benefits.

Yeast extract (Marmite) is salty but spread sparingly, it makes a useful carbohydrate-free alternative to jam in sandwiches and on toast.

What about additives?

With all the concern about healthy eating, many parents wonder if the amount of additives in processed foods is safe for their children. For most people, keeping a sensible balance between fresh foods and processed foods is all that is necessary. There are some children who are sensitive to some food additives but this is uncommon. If you are concerned about your own child, then discuss this with your dietitian or doctor.

Free foods

These foods contain negligible carbohydrate and are low in calories, and therefore may be eaten freely.

Fruits

Blackberries	Grapefruit	Red currants
Blackcurrants	Lemons	Rhubarb
Cranberries	Loganberries	
Gooseberries	Melon	

Vegetables

Artichokes	Celery	Olives
Asparagus	Courgettes	Onions
Aubergines	Cress	Peas, fresh or frozen
Beans, green and	Cucumber	Peppers
runner	Endive	Radishes
Beansprouts	Garlic	Spinach
Broccoli	Kale	Spring greens
Brussels sprouts	Leeks	Spring onions
Cabbage	Lettuce	Swede
Carrots	Marrow	Tomatoes
Cauliflower	Mushrooms	Turnips
Chicory	Mustard and cress	Watercress
Chinese cabbage	Okra	

Drinks

Bovril	Diabetic or sugar-free	Soup, clear
Coffee	or low-calorie	Tea
Mineral waters	squashes and fizzy	Tomato juice
Soda water	drinks	Water

Miscellaneous

Cocoa	Mustard	Sugar-free sweeteners
Curry powder	Pepper	(aspartame,
Flavourings	Pickles, clear	acesulfame K,
Gelatine	Soy sauce	saccharin)
Herbs	Spices	Tomato purée
Lemon juice	Stock cubes	Vinegar
Marmite		Worcester sauce

A weighty problem?

Overweight is the result of having an energy intake in excess of the body's needs. This can be caused by eating too much, taking less exercise, or by growth slowing down. All excess energy (calories) whether it comes from carbohydrates, fats or proteins is converted to fat and stored in the body.

Your child is unlikely to become overweight if he follows a diet rich in high-fibre carbohydrates and low in fats, avoids sugary foods and has a reasonable amount of exercise. But it is possible that when growth stops in adolescence, or if a child's growth slows down for a time, the previously adequate energy intake becomes surplus to requirements.

As with being overweight in any age group, it is much easier to deal with as soon as you notice it, rather than waiting until it has become a serious problem. It is advisable to discuss any dietary change with your dietitian and doctor to check what is best for your child's individual needs, especially if the insulin dose needs adjustment.

Adopting some or all of the measures suggested, the summary below may be all that is required to treat overweight. These changes do not affect the carbohydrate allowance of your child's diet and therefore the insulin requirement may not alter. For a growing child, the aim is to keep his weight steady rather than for him to lose weight. As he grows, his weight will become more in proportion to his height.

Carbohydrate exchange lists for adults, such as those produced by the British Diabetic Association, include calorie values of foods as well as the carbohydrate count. These can be a useful guide if your child does have a weight problem.

A healthy diet for your diabetic child

Twelve points to remember:	If your child has a weight problem:
1. Keep to the carbohydrate allowances for each meal and snack.	No need to reduce these (unless specifically advised to do so by your dietitian).
2. Choose high-fibre carbohydrates where possible.	Important when slimming as they are more satisfying and usually lower in calories.
3. Avoid sugar and sugary foods and drinks (for exceptions, see pages 24–28 and 34). Substitute with sweeteners, sugar-free squashes where necessary.	Avoid diabetic chocolates, sweets, cakes and biscuits the fructose and sorbitol they contain have a similar calorie value to sugar.
4. Include at least 400 ml/14 fl oz semi-skimmed milk each day (whole milk if under five years).	Change to fresh skimmed milk. Keep to natural or low-sugar yoghurts.

continued

5. At two meals each day have one of the protein foods: meat, fish, eggs, cheese or pulses.

6. Emphasize low-fat choices such as fish, chicken, low-fat cheese.

7. Try a pulse dish as a meat alternative at least once a week, more often if possible.

8. Encourage a taste for a wide variety of vegetables and fruit.	Green and salad vegetables are especially low in calories. Have fresh fruit or tinned fruit in natural juice for desserts (keeping ice cream, double cream and diabetic puddings for very special occasions).
9. Grill rather than fry and use oil for cooking where necessary.	Avoid fried food (including chips) altogether.
10. Change to a polyunsaturated margarine or low-fat spread for everyday use.	Keep to a scraping on bread or crispbread.
11. Take care not to add excess salt in cooking or at the table.	
12. Keep crisps and nuts to no more than once a day. Take fruit juice at meal-times only.	Crisps and nuts are high in calories so allow for special treats only. Encourage water and sugar-free squash to drink.

Emergency food for a 'hypo'

Hypo' is the shortened form of hypoglycaemia, the medical term meaning a low blood level of glucose. This can happen if your child misses or delays a meal or snack or inadvertently has too little carbohydrate. It can also occur if he has more insulin than he needs, or after exercise.

The symptons can be sweating, shaking, dizziness or confusion and also hunger or nausea, visual disturbance, tingling round lips and tongue and uncharacteristic tantrums. They are caused by a reduced supply of glucose to the brain because the blood level is low. Symptoms vary from person to person but each diabetic soon learns the warning signs of his own hypo. As well as you and your child being familiar with these symptoms, it is very important that anyone else caring for your child learns how to recognize a hypo. This includes grandparents or other relatives, close friends, teachers, playgroup leaders, or child minders. As soon as your child is old enough, he should be aware of how to recognize and treat a hypo himself.

The treatment is to give immediately 10–20 g of quickly absorbable carbohydrate (1–2 exchanges) such as sugar or glucose or a sweetened drink. The following suggestions each contain 10 g carbohydrate (1 exchange):

Glucose tablets	3
Sugar or glucose powder	2 level tsp
Sugar cubes	2
Honey, syrup, jam	2 level tsp
Lucozade	50 ml/1½ fl oz
Cola*	100 ml/3½ fl oz
Lemonade or other fizzy drink*	150 ml/¼ pint
Milk	200 ml/7 fl oz
Fruit juice (unsweetened)	100 ml/3½ fl oz

* These are sweetened drinks, not sugar-free or diabetic versions

Two exchanges could be made up by adding one of the solids to the fluids, for example, 2 tsp sugar or glucose in milk or fruit juice.

Taking readily absorbed carbohydrate should restore the blood glucose level to normal quite quickly. However, if after 10 minutes there is no improvement, give another 10–20 g carbohydrate (1–2 exchanges). If a meal or snack is not due within 30 minutes give an additional 10–20 g carbohydrate in the form of a starchy food such as bread or biscuits.

Although sweets and chocolates contain quickly available carbohydrate, it is not advisable to give these to combat a hypo, particularly in younger children. A three- or four-year-old could very quickly learn the potential reward available simply by saying he 'feels funny'. Glucose tablets or powder are useful for children as they come into the category of medicine rather than normally forbidden foods.

Always make sure your child carries a supply of emergency carbohydrate with him, at school for example. Glucose tablets are by far the most convenient source to keep in his pocket. It would be wise to let his teacher and the school welfare officer have a packet too.

Parents are sometimes given a supply of glucagon, a hormone which, when injected, causes a rise in the blood glucose level. This may be prescribed by the doctor especially in the case of young children who may be uncooperative or unable to swallow glucose during a hypo. When the child has recovered sufficiently, 20 g starchy carbohydrate should be given.

Extra food for exercise

Plenty of exercise is good for any child and there is no reason why diabetes should prevent your child enjoying all types of activity and sport.

The body needs extra energy for exercise and this may mean eating extra carbohydrate (even though the insulin dose is not increased). The amount needed will depend on the type and duration of the activity and may vary with each individual. You will soon find your own child's needs. Monitoring his blood glucose levels will help you decide.

Everyday activity
Regular normal exercise, such as playing, walking or cycling to school, needs no extra carbohydrate. The energy for this should be provided by the day's meals and snacks.

Extra activity
Your child must take additional carbohydrate for extra activities or sport. This activity falls into two categories: prolonged exercise (eg, football) and very strenuous exercise (usually shorter but more intense).

Prolonged exercise Here extra carbohydrate is needed in a slowly absorbed form (ie, starchy food) to cover the duration of the activity. Exercise in this category would include gym, ballet, football and other team games.

Try giving an extra 10–20 g carbohydrate (1–2 exchanges) at first, but increase this if blood sugar levels are too low. This must be taken just before the activity or with the preceding meal or snack, but remember it is extra to the usual carbohydrate amount. Suitable foods would be fruit (eg, 1 apple, 1 banana), crisps, 1 digestive biscuit, 2 wholewheat crackers or crispbread, 2 tbsp raisins or half a high-fibre crunchy bar.

Strenuous exercise For short, intense bursts of strenuous activity or for heavy exercise your child needs even more carbohydrate and in a quickly absorbable form (ie, sugar-based). You may find that he needs not only to eat beforehand but also afterwards, or even during.

Exercise in this category would include competitive athletics or swimming, judo and rowing. Most of these activities tend to apply to the older child.

Your child should take at least 20 g carbohydrate (2 exchanges) beforehand in a readily absorbable form, eg, chocolate-coated biscuit (eg, 1 Penguin, 2 Jaffa cakes); funsize Mars bar or Twix (1 finger) or KitKat (2 fingers); 1 glass cola or lemonade (sweetened type); 4 squares ordinary chocolate.

A larger amount of carbohydrate may be necessary at the next meal depending on the extent of the activity.

If strenuous exercise becomes regular, such as on an 'action holiday', your child may need to reduce his insulin dose as well as increasing the amount of daily carbohydrate. This extra should be taken as high-fibre and starchy foods (but with quickly absorbable carbohydrate available as a back-up). It is advisable to discuss these possible changes with your doctor or dietitian before the holiday, or regarding any particularly demanding sport such as running a marathon.

Every child is an individual and you may find certain activities need more extra carbohydrate, some less or none at all. Your child's blood glucose levels are the best guide on this.

Whatever the activity, make sure your child has some emergency carbohydrate such as glucose tablets on his person (not left in the changing room!) to take in case of hypoglycaemia.

Replacement food for illness

All children are ill occasionally and depending on the illness, their appetite may be affected. They may even be off their food for several days. If this happens, it is most important to continue with the daily insulin dose; in fact the need for insulin is frequently increased during illness, especially if the child has a fever. It is therefore essential that a regular supply of carbohydrate is maintained to prevent hypoglycaemia. Always consult your doctor if you are concerned about your child's condition or if it does not improve quickly.

When you child has lost his appetite, small frequent snacks of light food may be more acceptable than meals at the normal times. Make sure you achieve the usual total amount of daily carbohydrate. Remember to concentrate on giving foods that contain carbohydrate rather than free foods. Your child may be able to manage small amounts of breakfast cereal and milk, jam or honey sandwiches, biscuits, crackers or even crisps. Alternatively, milky drinks and puddings, ice cream, fruit yoghurt or ordinary jelly may be more suitable.

You can give an extra 10 g carbohydrate (1 exchange) by adding 2 tsp sugar or glucose to milky drinks, fruit juice, custard and blancmange. Jam or honey are pleasant in natural yoghurt or milk puddings. Baby foods and rusks softened in milk may be useful for young children.

If your child is nauseated or has a very sore throat, a few mouthfuls of sweetened fluid (eg, Lucozade, squash, cola, lemonade or glucose in water) every 15–20 minutes should maintain the blood glucose level. He may find it easier to drink with a straw. If feeling sick, fizzy drinks like Lucozade may be more acceptable when de-fizzed.

During a bout of diarrhoea or vomiting, only give sweetened fluids or ordinary jelly. Afterwards it is wise to introduce solid foods slowly, especially the high-fibre ones. Concentrate on the carbohydrates from the amber section (see page 10) like white bread, low-fibre cereals, white rice, mashed potatoes, for a day or so. Your child can return to eating his high-fibre diet once his digestive system is back to normal.

The following suggestions may be useful during illness (see also emergency carbohydrate list (page 25) and list of carbohydrate exchanges (page 117) for further ideas).

Fluids Each contains 10 g carbohydrate (1 exchange)

Lucozade	50 ml/1½ fl oz
Fruit juice	100 ml/3½ fl oz
Milk	200 ml/7 fl oz
Cola*	100 ml/3½ fl oz
Lemonade or other fizzy drink *	150 ml/¼ pint
Soup, thick or cream variety	200 ml/7 fl oz
Fruit squash (before dilution)*	35 ml/1¼ fl oz

* These are sweetened drinks, not sugar-free or diabetic versions

Be careful to measure these concentrated carbohydrate foods precisely using an accurate fluid measure or measuring spoons (available from the British Diabetic Association).

Semi-solid foods Each contains 20 g carbohydrate (2 exchanges)

Ice cream	2 scoops (100 g/3½ oz)
Fruit yoghurt	1 small carton
Natural yoghurt	1 small carton with 2 level tsp honey or jam
Milky drink	200 ml/7 fl oz milk with 2 tsp Ovaltine, Horlicks, Bournvita
Milk pudding	200 ml/7 fl oz milk with 1 tbsp custard powder, cornflour or pudding cereal
Jelly, ordinary	¼ of jelly made up to 1 pint or 3 jelly cubes
Rusk	1 Liga, 1 Oster, or ½ Farley's softened in 200 ml/7 fl oz milk

Poor diabetic control

A consistently high level of glucose can occur if a child is eating too much carbohydrate, having inadequate insulin or a reduced amount of activity. It can also happen due to illness or emotional stress. If this persists, the child will start to show the symptoms of diabetes (thirst, etc,) which could eventually lead to a diabetic coma. Consult your doctor without delay if your child's blood glucose levels are regularly too high, so that the treatment can be corrected.

From toddlers to teens

The age at which a child may develop diabetes varies greatly. If you are the parent of a newly diagnosed diabetic, you may be having to adjust the lifestyle of a child of any age, from toddler to teenager. Remember that many of the difficulties you encounter apply to non-diabetic children as well: the toddler whose mouth clamps firmly shut at the sight of food; the school child who hates to be different from his classmates; the rebellious teenager who rejects his parent's advice. Food is a very emotional subject and most children find the meal table an ideal battleground for fighting for independence.

When it is vital to eat the required amount of carbohydrate or to avoid tempting sweets, it is particularly difficult to react calmly when this is met with resistance. The art is trying to get a balance between insisting that dietary observance is important and yet not being over-protective so that your child feels like an invalid.

In general, children seem much better than adults at accepting and coping with a long-term condition like diabetes. You may be surprised at how quickly even a young child will learn the carbohydrate exchanges of common foods and the foods to be avoided. It is also easier for a child to 'lose his sweet tooth' than an adult.

Meeting other parents of diabetic children can be a tremendous support and encouragement. Find out about your local British Diabetic Association or hospital group.

The pre-school child

It is possible to have a greater control over what your child eats up to the age of five because most meals are taken at home. Most small children tend to have the advantage of fairly regular meals, snacks and bedtimes.

Getting a young child to eat up the food on his plate can be a problem, especially if it is the carefully measured carbohydrate food that he will not finish. It is best not to be too eager to replace that uneaten potato with some fruit or dessert to make up the carbohydrate. They will soon catch on! Encourage your child to finish the main meal but try to be nonchalant about it rather than over anxious. If gentle cajoling does not work, it may be better to meet halfway and replace the carbohydrate needed with bread rather than dessert.

In these early years, lay the foundations for a high-fibre, low-fat diabetic diet but remember that young children may not have the capacity for too much bulk. The priority is the correct amount of carbohydrate for good diabetic control. The main aims with this age group should be to avoid sugary foods, to encourage eating wholemeal bread and cereals, and to keep fried foods to a minimum. Skimmed milk is not recommended for children under five (unless advised for a weight problem); use whole milk.

Make sure that relatives, close friends, child-minders, play-group or nursery teachers know about your child's dietary needs. Beware of kindly visitors arriving with sweets.

The child at school

Once a child goes to school, he begins to take over some of the responsibility for caring for himself. He will have to be responsible for his meals and snacks during the time spent at school. As with all aspects of self-care, patient explanation and encouragement at home is the answer.

For school lunch, choosing between packed lunches or school meals is a matter of personal choice. Most school canteens will make special arrangements for a diabetic diet, for example, by providing fresh fruit for dessert. However, some school menus include a high proportion of convenience foods which tend to be higher in fat, such as chips, sausages and pies, and you may prefer to provide a more suitable meal in a packed lunch. Sending food from home at least ensures that the portions are already measured for your child, useful for a young child or newly diagnosed diabetic. Cafeteria systems operate in some schools and the older child may prefer to choose his diabetic meal from these.

Your child will also need to take food for midmorning and afternoon snacks. If these are carried together with the packed lunch, make sure the snacks and meal are wrapped separately to avoid confusion. The timing of the mid-afternoon snack may need some thought; it may suit one child in the afternoon playtime, while another could wait until getting home from school.

Children are very sensitive to their classmates' comments and may feel 'different' if they have to have a snack when no-one else does. Make sure the snack food you give causes least embarrassment – fruit, crisps or biscuits may be preferable to a sandwich. Find out the days on which sports or exercise are taken and provide an extra snack. Make sure your child understands the necessity of carrying glucose tablets at all times.

It is very important that the head teacher, class teacher and welfare officer are fully briefed about your child's needs. It is usual for your dietitian to contact the school and supply them with necessary information. The British Diabetic Association also produces a pack for teachers. It will be helpful to make sure the class teacher and/or welfare officer have a packet of glucose tablets and that they know how much carbohydrate your child needs at lunch, snacks and before exercise. It is equally important that the staff recognize that your child's condition will not prevent him from participating fully in games and other activities.

From school age your child will start to visit friends and go to parties without you. These are good opportunities for him to learn to take more responsibility for his diet. It may be wise to brief the friend's mother on suitable foods as well. Parties are dealt with in more detail on page 32.

The teenager

By the time a diabetic reaches his teens, he will be assuming much more responsibility for his diabetes and should be encouraged to do so. However, as in all other aspects of life, the parents should have overall responsibility.

Adolescence can be a time of rebellion and this may include a rejection of diabetic rules, such as eating unsuitable foods. This is not at all unusual and though worrying for the parent, it may be a crucial step in your child's personal acceptance of his condition. Like any rebelliousness and disobedience, it needs firm but sensitive handling. Make sure you are giving a reasonable amount of freedom of dietary choice suitable for your child's age. Consistent breaking of the diet may bring a lesson in itself when the child feels the effects of high blood glucose levels.

Severe and long-term rebellion needs medical help. In fact, a teenager who is rejecting parental authority may respond to advice from a caring outsider like your doctor, health visitor, social worker, church contact or friend of the family.

The teenage years bring more social eating with friends – for example, in hamburger and pizza bars, at parties and discos. Make sure your child is familiar with the carbohydrate values of foods he is likely to encounter. A less regular lifestyle is more common at this age – staying up late, lying in at weekends. While allowing a certain amount of flexibility, it is important that regular control of the diabetes is maintained. For example, it is wise not to delay the morning insulin injection and breakfast by more than an hour.

Above all, whatever his age, encourage your child not to use diabetes as an excuse for not taking part in activities or for bad behaviour. All children have their 'off' days but your own knowledge of your child should help you to distinguish between an oncoming hypo and being naughty.

On the positive side, your child has an advantage over many children in learning to eat a healthy diet and to cope with self-discipline.

Holidays, travel and diet

There is no reason why any holiday need be considered unsuitable for a diabetic child, including travel abroad. However, thoughtful planning beforehand will make an important difference to your trip.

Accommodation
Although a self-catering holiday means you have more control over the meals, staying in a hotel or guest house need not pose problems. Many family hotels in the UK cater for special diets. Notify them of your child's needs before going. It may also be worth mentioning that prompt table service would be desirable (though this tends to be more of a problem abroad).

If taking a foreign holiday, do not be intimidated by the thought of coping with unusual and different foods. Most countries have a staple carbohydrate food as part of the meal, eg, pasta, rice or bread. Take a comprehensive exchange list with you and if necessary diet scales to weigh foods you are not sure about.

In hotels and restaurants, the simpler meals are easier to analyse mentally than a complicated dish. Remember there is no carbohydrate in any type of meat, fish, eggs or cheese, while most vegetables have a very low content. Go for fresh fruit (washed carefully) or ice cream for dessert. Make sure you find sugar-free drinks for your child. If you buy natural fruit juices, check they are unsweetened. It is advisable to take sensible steps to reduce the risk of a stomach upset by making sure your child always drinks bottled water and avoids reheated or suspect dishes.

Children are nearly always more active on holiday so extra carbohydrate may be needed especially before swimming or long walks.

Holidays without parents
If the school teachers are agreeable, then a diabetic child should be able to cope with a school trip provided he is responsible enough to look after his own diet and injections. Remind him of the necessity of carrying glucose tablets at all times and taking extra carbohydrate for exercise. It would be wise to ask one teacher to be specifically briefed on your child's needs.

The British Diabetic Association runs holidays for diabetic children where, in addition to an enjoyable programme of activities, they can learn more about coping with their condition. The BDA also organize family weekends especially aimed at the new diabetic.

Travelling
The day of travel needs careful planning too. Whether it includes a flight or merely a long car journey, remember to take extra carbohydrate supplies, such as sandwiches, biscuits, fruit and crisps just in case meals are delayed. Make sure that the emergency glucose tablets are easy to find; keep them in pockets or in bags that are always near you. When flying, emergency rations and extra snacks should be kept in your hand luggage (along with insulin and syringes), not stowed away in the hold.

Not all the in-flight meals may be suitable for your child so, again, the extra supplies will come in handy. Ask for water if there are no suitable drinks available or bring your own (eg, small container of undiluted sugar-free squash).

When flying long distances east or west, the time change may mean an increase or reduction in the insulin dose and the number of meals needed for that day. It is best to discuss adjustments for a long journey like this with your own doctor and/or dietitian.

If travelling involves an early start, give your child a snack of 10–20 g carbohydrate (1–2 exchanges) on rising, then insulin and breakfast at the usual time. Similarly, a late night may mean giving another snack before bed in addition to the usual evening snack.

Remember it is preferable to err on the side of being over-generous with the carbohydrate to avoid the risk of a hypo while travelling. A hypo can be brought on by a change in routine or excitement in addition to the effects of an early start or a late night, travel delays or forgotten snacks.

If your child is prone to travel sickness, take the precaution of giving an anti-travel sickness medicine beforehand (your doctor will recommend a suitable brand). If vomiting still occurs, counteract this with sips of sweetened fluids.

Parties

Children's parties are normally held in the afternoon, often with the party tea being taken earlier than usual. As this is a special occasion, allow your child an extra 10–20 g carbohydrate (1–2 exchanges) in addition to the afternoon snack allowance. This will probably be compensated for by the extra activity and games. It is most inadvisable to give less carbohydrate at lunch time in order to save it for the afternoon allowance.

Giving parties
If it is your child's birthday party, make sure that everything you supply is suitable for him and let the other children fit in. For example, provide sugar-free squash for everyone; concentrate on savoury foods, such as crisps, nuts and dips; serve sugar-free jelly (made from squash and gelatine) or blancmange, fruit and ice cream. Make sandwiches and other nibbles in standard portions (eg, 1 exchange or less) and let your child know the carbohydrate value. The recipe section (page 107) gives lots of ideas for party food and suitable birthday cakes and icings. Novelty cakes need not rely on sugary decorations and piped icing. They can be made in a variety of shapes, eg, numbers, trains, or teddy bears (specially shaped baking tins can be hired from some kitchen supply shops), or decorated with models or pictures of a favourite television or story character.

Going to parties
If your child is going to a party without you, make sure he knows how much carbohydrate he is allowed. He should be able to make sensible guesses as to the carbohydrate value of the foods available, but warn him that the squash and jellies are unlikely to be sugar-free. Let him take his favourite sugar-free drink with him. It would be sensible to brief the organizer of the party of your child's dietary needs, so that sweets and lollies are not given for prizes or packed in his party bag to take home (suggest nuts or dried fruit instead or preferably a non-edible gift or prize). Although the birthday cake is best avoided at the party, a slice is usually given to take home. This could then be incorporated into the next meal's carbohydrate allowance, avoiding the icing.

Special food for diabetics

Sweeteners

There are a variety of sugar-free sweeteners available: intense sweeteners which can be used for sweetening drinks, fruit and milk puddings, and bulk sweeteners for use in baking biscuits and cakes. It is best to encourage your child to avoid added sweetening in tea, coffee and breakfast cereals, to use the intense sweeteners for 'sharp' fruits, desserts and puddings, and to keep the intake of foods containing bulk sweeteners to a minimum.

Intense sweeteners The three main intense sweeteners available are aspartame, saccharin and acesulfame K. They have a high sweetening power so are used in very small amounts. They also contain no carbohydrate and have a negligible calorie value. In the small quantities used, they are regarded as safe for use in children's diets (although aspartame is avoided in the rare condition phenylketonuria).

All three sweeteners are marketed in tablet form: aspartame (Canderel), saccharin (Hermesetas, Boots Shapers, Sweetex, Natrena), acesulfame K (Hermesetas Gold, Sweetex Plus, Diamin). These are usually used for sweetening hot drinks. Saccharin is available as a liquid sweetener (Hermesetas, Sweetex). This is convenient for sweetening stewed fruit, custards, milk puddings and other desserts. The powder forms of aspartame (Canderel Spoonful, Boots Shapers, Sweetex) and saccharin (Hermesetas Sprinkle Sweet) are useful for sprinkling on fruit or cereals. These powders contain small amounts of lactose (milk sugar) or maltodextrin (a type of starch) which add a minimal amount of carbohydrate and calories. Do not use powder sweeteners which contain sucrose. When cooking, remember that the sweetness of both saccharin and aspartame is reduced if added to very hot foods, so let them cool slightly first.

Bulk sweeteners As well as its ability to sweeten, sugar (or sucrose) gives bulk and texture in cakes, jams and confectionery. When trying to make diabetic versions of these foods, it is impossible to use an intense sweetener so bulk sweeteners are used instead. There are two main bulk sweeteners: sorbitol and fructose or fruit sugar (Dietade).

Remember that these substances should be used with caution in the diabetic diet. Although they contain no glucose, they both have a similar energy (calorie) value to sugar and therefore add unnecessary calories to the diet. Sorbitol has a laxative effect if taken to excess and can cause flatulence. The metabolism of fructose is not completely understood and in some circumstances it can cause a rise in the blood glucose level.

For these reasons, bulk sweeteners should be avoided by any diabetic with a weight problem, and it is advised by the British Diabetic Association that all diabetics should have no more than 25 g/¾ oz of one or a combination of bulk sweeteners in any one day. Remember this means both home-cooked foods and bought products containing fructose or sorbitol.

Nevertheless fructose and sorbitol have a use in baking cakes and some biscuits, and as an ingredient in jams, marmalade, chocolate and sweets. Keep these foods to a minimum in the diet. Never use bulk sweeteners for sweetening fruit, cereals or milk puddings where intense sweeteners would be just as effective.

When using fructose or sorbitol you do not need to count their carbohydrate content, provided you keep within the BDA recommended maximum.

Useful proprietary foods for children

It is perfectly possible to have a varied diabetic diet with only very small amounts of special 'diabetic' foods. These proprietary products are not a necessity and do tend to be more expensive than non-diabetic varieties.

Sugar-free fruit squashes, cordials and fizzy drinks (bottled and canned, eg, Diet-coke) are probably the most useful in a diabetic child's diet. These are normally sweetened with aspartame (Nutrasweet) or saccharin and may be labelled for diabetics, slimmers or as low calorie (eg, Boots, Roses brands). Pure lemon juice (PLJ), slimline drinks and mineral waters are also suitable.

Tinned fruit for diabetics is normally sweetened with saccharin and many varieties of ordinary canned fruit are now available in natural juice.

Slimmers' fruit yoghurts (see page 20) are very useful as they are as low or lower in carbohydrate than natural yoghurt.

Diabetic jams and marmalade contain sorbitol so spread thinly on bread and toast.

There are a variety of sweets (pastilles, fruit drops, peppermints, chewing gum) and chocolates available for diabetics. These all contain sorbitol or fructose so make sure they are kept for treats rather than for regular consumption.

Other diabetic products include fancy biscuits, cake mix, jelly and instant desserts. These normally contain sorbitol or fructose and tend to be expensive. It is better to buy suitable 'ordinary' biscuits and to make your own cakes and puddings where possible.

Make sure your child has no more than the BDA maximum of 25 g /³/₄ oz of bulk sweeteners in any one day.

Use of sugar in your child's diet

While it is important to avoid all unnecessary sugar, there are times when its use would improve a recipe or enhance the palatability of the high-fibre diet. Recent studies have led to a BDA recommendation that a modest amount of sugar can be allowed for a diabetic provided it is taken with or after a high fibre meal. Sugar should never be used where an intense sweetener would do just as well. However, when a bulk sweetener is required, such as in baking cakes, sugar (or sucrose) gives a better result than fructose and is less expensive. Sucrose is the chemical term for sugar used in the home, i.e. white sugar (granulated, castor, icing) and all types of brown sugar. The BDA have recommended that an adult diabetic could take up to a maximum of 25g of sucrose per day. The amount for a child depends on their age and individual needs, so check this with you dietitian or doctor before using sugar in recipes or buying cake etc. The sugar must be counted as part of the carbohydrate allowance. It should be used instead of, not in addition to, the allowance of fructose. Remember that sugar gives no other nutrients apart from carbohydrate and is therefore best kept to a minimum in any child's diet.

For recipes in this book requiring a bulk sweetener, a choice between sugar (sucrose) or fructose is given. The analyses include the calorie value and carbohydrate content for sugar, but if fructose is used the carbohydrate content is not counted.

THE RECIPES:
INTRODUCTION

The recipes in this book have been specifically designed for the family cook who has to cater for a diabetic child. Most of the recipes are equally suitable for everyday family meals; indeed some of them are probably familiar favourites, albeit adapted as necessary in certain cases. Hopefully this means that they are recipes that children will like and will eat.

All the recipes are designed both to increase the amount of fibre in the diet and to minimize the fat content. They have also been nutritionally analyzed to make carbohydrate exchange calculations easier (see below).

The majority of the dishes described are for everyday meals, snacks and drinks. The emphasis throughout is on speed and ease of preparation, as time and energy are limited for most people preparing such food. There are also some recipes which are intended for celebrations, such as a birthday, when one may want to provide a special treat. It is important to take extra care when measuring the portions of these.

Weights and measures
Both metric and imperial measurements are given in the recipes. Metric measurements were used both for testing the recipes and calculating the nutritional analyses. For convenience and speed in the kitchen, small quantities of ingredients are frequently given in tablespoon measures. The tablespoon measurement used throughout refers to a level 15 ml tablespoon. Similarly, teaspoons are equivalent to a level 5 ml measure. Standard measuring spoons are obtainable from the British Diabetic Association. Australian users should remember that as their tablespoon has been converted to 20 ml, and is therefore larger than the tablespoon measurement used in the recipes in this book, they should use 3 x 5 ml tsp where 1 x 15 ml tbsp is specified.

Nutritional analyses precede each recipe. Carbohydrate has been rounded off to the nearest 10 g and each 10 g is referred to as 1 exchange. Most recipes have portions of 10 g (1 exchange) or multiples thereof. Occasionally a portion may have only 5 g carbohydrate (0.5 exchange).

Where a portion has less than 1 g carbohydrate, the value is stated as negligible.

Calories (kcal) have been rounded off to the nearest 10.

Fibre, protein and fat content have been rounded off to the nearest gram.

Ingredients
Certain ingredients have been used as standard in all the recipes. These have been chosen to promote good health and a balanced diet and the cooking methods have been adapted where necessary. We recommend that you should use the following in your cooking:

- Wholemeal (also called wholewheat) cereal products, breads and pasta.

- 100 per cent wholemeal flour in all baking. The cooking methods described for wholemeal pastry and cakes have been devised particularly to combat any heaviness in the finished.product.

- Brown rice in savoury and sweet dishes.

- Pulses, ie, dried peas, beans and lentils.

- Semi-skimmed milk. This has a reduced fat content but retains essential fat-soluble vitamins A and D.

- Skimmed milk natural yoghurt. This can be used as a substitute for cream in many dishes and also replaces commercial, sweetened yoghurts.

- Skimmed milk soft cheese. Sometimes called fromage blanc or quark. This is also useful as a substitute for cream in savoury or sweet dishes.

- Hard cheeses. A tasty mature Cheddar is recommended for cooking as smaller amounts are required for a good flavour, thus helping to reduce the fat content. When a hard cheese is used for sandwiches or salads, a lower-fat variety such as Edam or Gouda is recommended.

- Polyunsaturated oils, fats and margarine are recommended for all cooking and spreading purposes.

- Lean meat. Trim off any visible fat and drain off the fat after frying minced meat. Always buy low-fat varieties of sausages and sausagemeat.

- Leave the skin on potatoes in all dishes except those requiring mashed potato. Similarly, leave the skin on other fruits and vegetables wherever possible.

- Herbs are used frequently in the recipes to add natural flavour. The quantities given generally refer to dried herbs, although fresh ones are always preferable if available. If you are using fresh herbs, add three times the amount given for dried.

- The use of raw eggs is not recommended. Use pasteurised dried egg white in all recipes which need it.

- Sugar-free sweeteners are recommended for use in cooking, ie, saccharin, acesulfame K and aspartame. Liquid saccharin is specified in the recipes most often as it is easier to blend and does not lose its sweetness during cooking at high temperatures. Aspartame powder sweetener is preferred for any dishes which do not require cooking. Some recipes include castor sugar (sucrose) as a bulk sweetener but this has only been used where necessary to give an acceptable result. Fructose may be used as an alternative to castor sugar if preferred. Energy values and carbohydrate exchanges are given for both.

Servings

Most of the recipes provide either four or six servings of an average size. Carbohydrate exchange values are per serving as stated in each recipe unless otherwise indicated.

Obviously, the appetite of a child varies greatly, according to his age, state of health and growth rate. The balancing of carbohydrate exchanges has to be calculated accordingly.

Fast food
Cooking for children often seems to demand cooking of the 'fast food' variety. Eating sensibly does not preclude such fast food provided some thought has been given to advance preparation.
Here are some ideas and tips to enable meals to be put together in a hurry:

- Cooked brown rice and pulses can be stored for several days in a refrigerator and used to prepare nutritious salads, soups, stir-fries, burgers or fritters quickly, with other fresh ingredients. Cooked brown rice and pulses can also be frozen, making bulk cooking and freezing a time- and fuel-saving operation. Allow 2 hours for defrosting.

- Any burgers in the recipes may be individually frozen and stored in a plastic bag in the freezer. One or two can then be removed at any time and cooked from frozen. Prepare double or treble quantities and freeze them.

- Individual portions of puddings and desserts, especially fruit mousses and ice creams, can be frozen and defrosted more quickly than large quantities. Freeze these in yoghurt pots or polystyrene cups.

- Ice-cube trays or bags are invaluable for freezing tablespoonfuls of unsweetened fruit purées such as apricot, prune, blackcurrant or apple. These can then be thawed rapidly and used to flavour natural yoghurt or milk shakes, or to serve with ice cream or milk puddings.

Cooking pulses
An enormous variety of pulses is now available in supermarkets, as well as in specialist food shops and health food stores. Canned ready-cooked pulses are convenient and a useful standby, but check the labels to see if sugar has been added. If so, rinse the beans thoroughly.

Dried pulses are much cheaper but many people are put off by the long cooking and soaking times involved. It is true that all pulses benefit from soaking for 5–8 hours in plenty of cold water. After either a hot or a cold soak the pulses need to be rinsed and then cooked in fresh water. If beans, especially red beans are not cooked thoroughly, they may cause severe food poisoning. To avoid this, make sure that they are covered by their own depth again in water. Bring the pan to the boil and boil hard for at least 10 minutes, then turn the heat down and simmer more gently for the appropriate cooking time as given in table overleaf.

Pulses can also be cooked in a pressure cooker and this reduces the cooking times considerably, which is particularly useful for those varieties requiring the longer cooking times. It is, however, easy to overcook pulses in a pressure cooker, so it is necessary to keep a sharp eye on the cooking times.

Average cooking times are given in the table as there will be variations according to the age of the pulses, older ones being harder and drier.

See table overleaf

Type of pulse	Average cooking time	Pressure cooking time
Split red lentils: unsoaked	20–30 minutes	5–10 minutes

Split peas:
  unsoaked
  soaked
	45–60 minutes
	25–30 minutes
		15 minutes
		10 minutes

Continental lentils:
  unsoaked
  soaked
	1–1½ hours
	45–60 minutes
		20–30 minutes
		15–20 minutes

Black-eyed beans	25–30 minutes	10–15 minutes
Mung beans	25–30 minutes	10–15 minutes
Field beans	30–60 minutes	15–20 minutes
Flageolet beans	30–60 minutes	15–20 minutes
Butter beans	45–60 minutes	15–20 minutes
Red kidney beans	1–1¼ hours	20–25 minutes
Aduki beans	1–1½ hours	25–30 minutes
Black beans	1–1½ hours	25–30 minutes
Cannellini beans	1–1½ hours	25–30 minutes
Haricot beans	1–1½ hours	25–30 minutes
Chick peas	1–2 hours	35–40 minutes
Soya beans	2–3 hours	1 hour

BREAKFASTS

Eggy bread

Serves 2

Each serving: 140 kcal/600 kJ, 10 g (1 exchange) carbohydrate, 3 g fibre, 7 g protein, 7 g fat

1 egg
4 tbsp semi-skimmed milk
seasoning

2 x 25 g/³/₄ oz slices wholemeal bread
polyunsaturated oil for frying

Beat the egg with the milk and season. Pour the egg mixture over the bread on a flat dish or plate. Turn the bread several times to soak up the egg. Heat a little oil in a frying pan, and fry the slices briskly for 2–3 minutes on each side. Serve immediately.

Bacon scramble

Serves 1

Total recipe: 210 kcal/890 kJ, 10 g (1 exchange) carbohydrate, 3 g fibre, 16 g protein, 11 g fat

1 rasher lean bacon, chopped
1 egg
1 tbsp semi-skimmed milk

seasoning
1 x 25 g/³/₄ oz slice wholemeal toast

Put the bacon into a heavy pan and cook slowly at first to release the fat. Turn up the heat and crisp the bacon. Drain off any excess fat. Whisk the egg with the milk and seasoning. Pour over the bacon and stir over a low heat until the egg is softly scrambled. Serve on hot toast.

Cheesy oat fritters

Makes 10

Each fritter: 90 kcal/390 kJ, 10 g (1 exchange) carbohydrate, negligible fibre, 4 g protein, 5 g fat

50 g/1¹/₂ oz rolled oats
50 g/1¹/₂ oz wholemeal flour
1 egg
300 ml/¹/₂ pint semi-skimmed milk

¹/₂ tsp dry mustard
seasoning
50 g/1¹/₂ oz Cheddar cheese, grated
polyunsaturated oil for frying

Mix together the oats, flour, mustard, and seasoning. Make a well in the centre and break the egg into it. Pour in a little of the milk. Begin mixing the egg into the flour and oats with a wooden spoon. Beat well and gradually add the remaining milk. Stir in the cheese. Heat a little oil in a frying pan and fry tablespoonfuls of the mixture. Allow the mixture to set and brown (3–4 minutes) before turning once. Serve immediately.

Banana crunch See photograph, page 49

Serves 2

Each serving: 140 kcal/580 kJ, 20 g (2 exchanges) carbohydrate, 2 g fibre, 9 g protein, 2 g fat

300 ml/¹/₂ pint natural yoghurt
1 small banana, sliced

15 g/¹/₂ oz wheatflakes, toasted
sugar-free sweetener to taste

Pour the yoghurt over the banana slices, sprinkle the wheatflakes on top and sweeten if necessary.

Tomato cheese toasts

Serves 2

Each serving: 140 kcal/590 kJ, 10 g (1 exchange) carbohydrate, 3 g fibre, 10 g protein, 5 g fat

2 x 25 g/³/₄ oz slices wholemeal
 bread
1 tomato, cut into small pieces

2 tbsp cottage cheese
25 g/³/₄ oz Cheddar cheese, grated

Toast the bread on one side. Mix the tomato with the cheeses. Spread the mixture on the untoasted side of the bread and grill for 2–3 minutes until the cheese melts and bubbles. Serve immediately.

Fishy toasts

Serves 2

Each serving: 220 kcal/930 kJ, 10 g (1 exchange) carbohydrate, 3 g fibre, 19 g protein, 10 g fat

1 tsp polyunsaturated oil
50 g/1¹/₂ oz cooked smoked
 fish (haddock or kipper), flaked
2 eggs, beaten
4 tbsp semi-skimmed milk

pepper
2 tbsp skimmed milk soft cheese
2 x 25 g/³/₄ oz slices wholemeal
 bread

Heat the oil in a saucepan, add the flaked fish and heat gently for 2 minutes. Add the eggs and milk, season with pepper and cook over a low heat, stirring continuously as the mixture thickens. When the eggs are cooked, stir in the cheese. Toast the bread on both sides and divide the fish mixture between the two slices. Serve immediately.

Breakfast kedgeree See photograph, page 49

Serves 2

Each serving: 180 kcal/740 kJ, 10 g (1 exchange) carbohydrate, negligible fibre, 11 g protein, 9 g fat

2 tsp polyunsaturated oil
1 tomato, chopped
50 g/1¹/₂ oz cooked smoked
 fish, flaked

100 g/3¹/₂ oz cooked brown rice
1 hard-boiled egg, chopped
pepper

Heat the oil in a frying pan and cook the chopped tomato for 1 minute. Add the fish and rice and stir over the heat to heat them through. Add the chopped egg, cook for 1–2 minutes, season with pepper and serve.

Yoghurt breakfast

Serves 2
Each serving: 140 kcal/610 kJ, 20 g (2 exchanges) carbohydrate, 2 g fibre, 10 g protein, 2 g fat

350 ml/12 fl oz natural yoghurt   *15 g/¹/₂ oz sultanas*
1 eating apple, chopped   *15 g/¹/₂ oz wheatgerm*

Mix all the ingredients together and serve.

SOUPS

Hearty bean soup   See photograph, page 50

Serves 4

Each serving: 160 kcal/670 kJ, 20 g (2 exchanges) carbohydrate, 8 g fibre, 7 g protein, 8 g fat

2 tbsp polyunsaturated oil
1 medium-sized onion, finely chopped
1 medium-sized carrot, diced
1 celery stalk, diced
100 g/3¹/2 oz aduki beans or red
   kidney beans, soaked in cold
   water overnight
1 clove garlic, crushed

400 g/14 oz chopped canned tomatoes
   and juice
1 bay leaf
¹/2 tsp dried thyme
¹/2 tsp dried basil
750 ml/1¹/4 pints water
seasoning

Heat the oil in a large saucepan and add the chopped onion, carrot and celery. Cover with a lid and cook slowly for 10–15 minutes, stirring occasionally. Add the drained beans and all the remaining ingredients except the seasoning. Bring the soup to the boil, cover and simmer for 1–1¹/4 hours until the beans are tender. Season to taste and serve. The soup can be frozen.

Leek soup

Serves 4

Each serving: 130 kcal/550 kJ, 10 g (1 exchange) carbohydrate, 2 g fibre, 5 g protein, 7 g fat

25 g/³/4 oz polyunsaturated margarine
1 onion, finely chopped
1 medium-sized potato, diced
2 leeks, finely chopped
black pepper

300 ml/¹/2 pint semi-skimmed milk
450 ml/³/4 pint chicken or vegetable
   stock
seasoning

Melt the margarine in a saucepan, toss the chopped vegetables in the fat and season with pepper. Cover with a lid and cook slowly for 5 minutes. Stir occasionally to prevent browning. Add the milk and stock. Bring to the boil and simmer for 20 minutes. Liquidize, process or purée the soup and season to taste.

Kidney soup

Serves 6

Each serving: 70 kcal/290 kJ, 5 g (0.5 exchange) carbohydrate, 1 g fibre, 7 g protein, 3 g fat

15 g/¹/2 oz polyunsaturated
   margarine

1 onion, finely chopped
200 g/7 oz ox kidney, diced

15 g/1½ oz wholemeal flour
750 ml/1¼ pints stock
400 g/14 oz canned tomatoes,
  chopped with juice

1 tsp dried mixed herbs
seasoning

Melt the margarine in a saucepan and fry the onion gently for 2–3 minutes. Add the kidney, turn up the heat and cook briskly to brown. Stir in the flour and cook for 1 minute before adding the stock, tomatoes, herbs and seasoning. Bring to the boil and simmer for 30 minutes. Liquidize or purée the soup before serving.

Celery soup

Serves 4
Each serving: 100 kcal/410 kJ, 10 g (1 exchange) carbohydrate, 2 g fibre, 4 g protein, 7 g fat

25 g/¾ oz polyunsaturated
  margarine
1 onion, finely chopped
5 celery stalks, finely chopped

300 ml/½ pint semi-skimmed
  milk
450 ml/¾ pint chicken or
  vegetable stock
seasoning

Melt the margarine in a saucepan and stir in the chopped vegetables. Cover with a lid and cook very gently for 10–15 minutes, stirring occasionally to prevent browning. Add the milk, stock and seasoning, bring to the boil and simmer gently for 20 minutes. Liquidize or purée the soup and adjust the seasoning to taste before serving.

Quick minestrone soup

Serves 4
Each serving: 90 kcal/390 kJ, 10 g (1 exchange) carbohydrate, 3 g fibre, 3 g protein, 5 g fat

25 g/¾ oz polyunsaturated
  margarine
1 onion, chopped
1 leek, chopped
1 carrot, diced
2 celery stalks, chopped
400 g/14 oz canned tomatoes,
  chopped with juice

450 ml/¾ pint stock or water
1 tsp dried oregano
½ tsp dried thyme
seasoning
15 g/1½ oz wholemeal pasta

Melt the margarine in a saucepan and toss the chopped vegetables until well coated in fat. Turn the heat down low, cover with a lid and cook for 10 minutes, stirring occasionally to prevent browning. Add the chopped tomatoes, stock or water, herbs and seasoning. Bring to the boil and simmer for 15 minutes. Add the pasta and cook for a further 15 minutes. Serve the soup with a light sprinkling of grated cheese, Parmesan or other.

Lettuce soup   See photograph, page 50

Serves 4

Each serving: 120 kcal/520 kJ, 10 g (1 exchange) carbohydrate, 1 g fibre, 4 g protein, 7 g fat

25 g/³/₄ oz polyunsaturated
  margarine
1 small onion, finely chopped
1 medium-sized potato, diced
8–10 large lettuce leaves (outer),
  shredded

black pepper
300 ml/¹/₂ pint semi-skimmed
  milk
450 ml/³/₄ pint chicken or
  vegetable stock

Melt the margarine in a saucepan and add the onion and potato. Stir to coat the vegetables in the fat, cover with a lid and 'sweat' over a low heat for 5 minutes. Add the shredded lettuce, stir well and cook, covered, for about 3 minutes or until the lettuce has shrunk. Season well with black pepper, add the milk and stock, bring to the boil and simmer for 20 minutes. Liquidize or process the soup, check the seasoning and serve.

Carrot and lentil soup   See photograph, page 50

Serves 4

Each serving: 80 kcal/330 kJ, 10 g (1 exchange) carbohydrate, 2 g fibre, 2 g protein, 5 g fat

25 g/³/₄ oz polyunsaturated
  margarine
¹/₂ small onion, finely chopped
200 g/7 oz carrots, diced

1 tsp dried thyme
15 g/¹/₂ oz red lentils
600 ml/1 pint stock or water
seasoning

Melt the margarine in a saucepan. Stir in the chopped onion and carrots until well coated with the fat. Cover with a lid and cook the vegetables very slowly for 10–15 minutes, stirring occasionally to prevent browning. Add the thyme, lentils and stock or water. Bring to the boil and simmer for 30 minutes until the carrots are tender. Season to taste. Liquidize or purée the soup if desired. This soup can be frozen in an airtight container.

SALADS

Green 'crunch' salad See photograph, page 59

Serves 4
Each serving: 130 kcal/530 kJ, 10 g (1 exchange) carbohydrate, 3 g fibre, 3 g protein, 10 g fat

250 g/9 oz Iceberg or other crisp lettuce, shredded
7.5 cm/3 in long piece cucumber sliced
50 g/1¹/2 oz green pepper, thinly sliced
100 g/3¹/2 oz green grapes, halved and seeded

2 celery stalks, sliced diagonally
25 g/³/4 oz toasted flaked almonds

Dressing
2 tbsp mayonnaise
4 tbsp natural yoghurt
seasoning

Assemble all the ingredients in a salad bowl. Combine the dressing ingredients. Just before serving, pour the dressing over the salad and toss well to coat everything.

Rainbow salad See photograph, page 59

Serves 3
Each serving: 60 kcal/230 kJ, 10 g (1 exchange) carbohydrate, 5 g fibre, 4 g protein, negligible fat

100 g/3¹/2 oz frozen peas
50 g/1¹/2 oz frozen sweetcorn
100 g/3¹/2 oz carrots, diced
2 tomatoes, chopped

5 spring onions, chopped
2 tbsp skimmed milk soft cheese
seasoning

Cook the frozen peas and sweetcorn for 3–5 minutes in boiling water. Drain and refresh in cold water. Mix all the ingredients together, seasoning to taste.

Red cabbage and pineapple salad See photograph, page 59

Serves 4
Each serving: 120 kcal/520 kJ, 10 g (1 exchange) carbohydrate, 3 g fibre, 3 g protein, 7 g fat

25 g/³/4 oz sultanas
200 g/7 oz pineapple, fresh or canned unsweetened
150 g/5 oz red cabbage, finely shredded
25 g/³/4 oz unsalted peanuts
1 tbsp chopped parsley

Dressing
1 tbsp polyunsaturated oil
2 tsp vinegar
¹/2 tsp French mustard
seasoning

Soak the sultanas for 1 hour in a little boiling water or juice from the pineapple. Place the pineapple, cabbage, peanuts, sultanas and parsley in a salad bowl.

Whisk the dressing ingredients with a fork and pour over the salad. Toss well and serve.

Apple slaw

Serves 4
Each serving: 100 kcal/420 kJ, 10 g (1 exchange) carbohydrate, 2 g fibre, 2 g protein, 5 g fat

2 dessert apples, cored and sliced
100 g/3¹/₂ oz white cabbage, shredded
50 g/1¹/₂ oz carrot, grated
15 g/¹/₂ oz sultanas

15 g/¹/₂ oz sesame seeds

Dressing
2 tbsp natural yoghurt
1 tbsp lemon juice
1 tbsp mayonnaise
seasoning

Prepare the salad ingredients, and place in a bowl. Mix together the dressing ingredients and pour over the salad. Stir well to coat everything. Sprinkle the sesame seeds over the top and serve.

Rice and lentil salad

Serves 4
Each serving: 160 kcal/650 kJ, 20 g (2 exchanges) carbohydrate, 3 g fibre, 6 g protein, 4 g fat

200 g/7 oz cooked brown rice
200 g/7 oz cooked green or brown
  lentils
2 tomatoes, chopped
2 celery stalks, chopped
7.5 cm/3 in long piece cucumber,
  chopped

1 tbsp chopped parsley

Dressing
1 tbsp polyunsaturated oil
1 tbsp lemon juice
¹/₂ tsp French mustard
seasoning

Combine all the ingredients in a salad bowl.

Whisk the dressing ingredients with a fork and pour over the salad. Stir and turn over carefully to disperse the dressing.

Prawn potato salad

Serves 4
Each serving: 240 kcal/1020 kJ, 20 g (2 exchanges) carbohydrate, 2 g fibre, 15 g protein, 13 g fat

400 g/14 oz cooked new potatoes,
  cut into 2.5 cm/1 in pieces
4 hard-boiled eggs, cut into
  2.5 cm/1 in pieces
100 g/3¹/₂ oz shelled prawns

Dressing
2 tbsp mayonnaise
2 tsp lemon juice
2 tbsp natural yoghurt
seasoning

2 tbsp snipped chives (to garnish)

Mix the potatoes and eggs with the prawns. Mix together the dressing ingredients, pour over the salad and toss gently. Garnish with the chives.

FISH AND MEAT DISHES

Salmon and rice bake

Serves 6
Each serving: 370 kcal/1540 kJ, 40 g (4 exchanges) carbohydrate, 5 g fibre, 21 g protein, 35 g fat

1 tbsp polyunsaturated oil
250 g/9 oz brown rice
750 ml/1¹/4 pints boiling water
¹/2 tsp mixed dried herbs
200 g/7 oz fresh or frozen peas
100 g/3¹/2 oz fresh or frozen green beans

300 g/7 oz canned salmon, drained and flaked
2 eggs
450 ml/³/4 pint semi-skimmed milk
100 g/3¹/2 oz Cheddar cheese, grated

Heat the oil in a heavy-based saucepan, add the rice and cook for 2 minutes, stirring continuously. Add the boiling water and herbs. Stir, then cover closely and cook over a very low heat for 45 minutes or until the rice is tender and the water has been absorbed. Mix the uncooked peas and beans into the cooked rice, together with the flaked salmon. Season well and transfer the mixture to an ovenproof dish. Preheat the oven to 190°C/375°F/gas 5. Beat the eggs with the milk and pour over the rice mixture. Sprinkle the cheese over the top and bake for 25–30 minutes until firm and golden.

Tuna spaghetti   See photograph, page 60

Serves 4
Each serving: 350 kcal/1480 kJ, 50 g (5 exchanges) carbohydrate, 9 g fibre, 24 g protein, 6 g fat

1 tbsp polyunsaturated oil
1 onion, finely chopped
1 tsp dried basil
50 g/1¹/2 oz mushrooms, chopped
400 g/14 oz canned tomatoes, chopped with juice

300 g/10¹/2 oz wholemeal spaghetti
200 g/7 oz canned tuna fish in brine, drained and flaked
seasoning

Heat the oil in a saucepan and soften the onion for 2–3 minutes. Add the basil and mushrooms and cook for a further 2–3 minutes. Add the tomatoes. Simmer the sauce, uncovered, for 30 minutes.

Cook the spaghetti in fast-boiling water for 10 minutes. Drain and mix with the flaked tuna and hot tomato sauce. Season and serve immediately.

Fish pie

Serves 4
Each serving: 400 kcal/1660 kJ, 40 g (4 exchanges) carbohydrate, 4 g fibre, 32 g protein, 11 g fat

500 g/1¼ lb cod or haddock
bay leaf
25 g/¾ oz polyunsaturated
margarine
seasoning
600 ml/1 pint semi-skimmed
milk
25 g/¾ oz wholemeal flour

50 g/1½ oz fresh or frozen
peas
50 g/1½ oz frozen sweetcorn
1 tbsp chopped parsley
1 tbsp lemon juice
600 g/1½ lb potatoes,
boiled and mashed with
2 tbsp natural yoghurt

Preheat the oven to 190°C/375°F/gas 5.
Put the fish into a frying pan with the bay leaf, margarine and seasoning. Pour over the milk. Bring to the boil, cover and simmer for 10 minutes. Lift out the fish and discard the bay leaf. Reserve the milk. Remove any skin and bones and flake the fish. Gradually whisk the flour into the cooled milk and heat slowly, whisking continuously until it boils and thickens. Simmer for 2 minutes. Add the peas, sweetcorn, flaked fish, parsley and lemon juice. Season to taste. Transfer to an ovenproof pie dish and top with the mashed potatoes. Bake for 20–30 minutes.

Tuna fish cakes

Makes 10
Each fish cake: 80 kcal/350 kJ, 10 g (1 exchange) carbohydrate, negligible fibre, 7 g protein, 4 g fat

200 g/7 oz canned tuna fish in
brine, drained
250 g/9 oz mashed potato
1 tbsp natural yoghurt
1 tbsp chopped parsley
2 tsp lemon juice

seasoning
1 egg, beaten
25 g/¾ oz fresh wholemeal
breadcrumbs
2 tbsp polyunsaturated oil for
frying

Mash the tuna with a fork, then mix it with the potato, yoghurt, parsley, lemon juice and seasoning. Divide the mixture into ten equal pieces and shape into cakes. Dip each cake into beaten egg, then breadcrumbs to coat. Shallow fry in a small amount of oil for 5 minutes on each side.
The uncooked fish cakes can be frozen. Open freeze and put into a polythene bag when frozen.

Opposite: Apricot milk shake (*top*, see page 101); Breakfast kedgeree (*centre*, see page 40); Herb scones (*bottom left*, see page 102); Banana crunch (*bottom right*, see page 40)

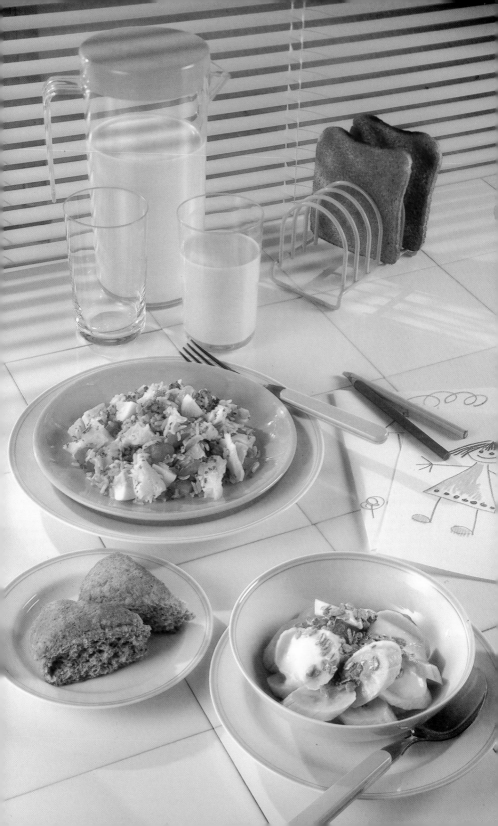

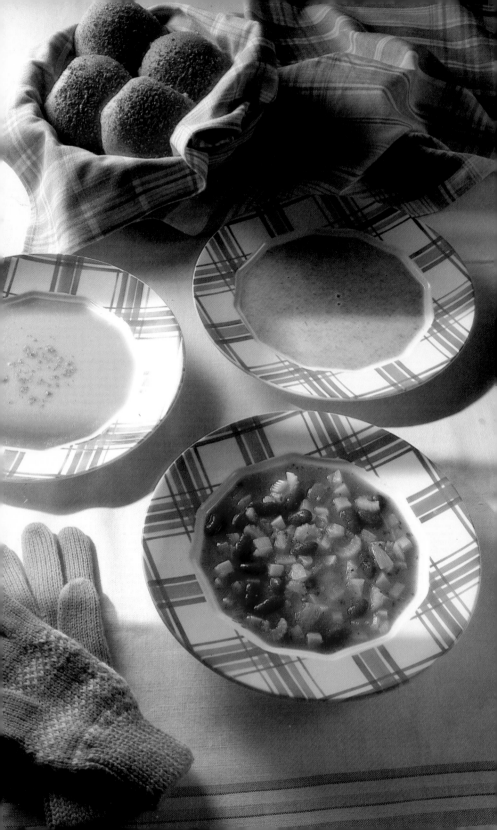

Chicken burgers

Makes 6
Each burger: 190 kcal/810 kJ, 10 g (1 exchange) carbohydrate, 2 g fibre, 18 g protein, 10 g fat

1 tbsp polyunsaturated
margarine
1 onion, finely chopped
350 g/12 oz cooked minced
chicken, (without skin)
75 g/2¹/2 oz fresh wholemeal
breadcrumbs
¹/2 tsp dried thyme
1 tbsp fresh chopped parsley

1 tsp tomato purée
seasoning
1 egg, beaten
polyunsaturated oil for frying

To coat
1 egg, beaten
25 g/3/4 oz fresh wholemeal
breadcrumbs

Melt the margarine and fry the onion gently until soft and transparent. Mix together the onion, chicken, breadcrumbs, herbs, tomato purée and seasoning. Add enough beaten egg to bind the mixture together. Divide the mixture into six portions and shape each one into a flat round cake. Dip each into beaten egg, then breadcrumbs and fry in a little oil for about 7 minutes on each side.

The burgers may be frozen before frying. Open freeze and then place in an airtight container when frozen.

Chicken pie

Serves 6
Each serving: 320 kcal/1350 kJ, 20 g (2 exchanges) carbohydrate, 3 g fibre, 22 g protein, 17 g fat

1 tbsp polyunsaturated oil
1 onion, finely chopped
1 clove garlic, crushed
100 g/3¹/2 oz mushrooms,
sliced
25 g/3/4 oz wholemeal flour
300 ml/¹/2 pint semi-skimmed
milk
300 ml/¹/2 pint chicken stock

¹/2 tsp dried thyme
1 tbsp chopped parsley
400 g/14 oz cooked chicken
meat (without skin), cubed
50 g/1¹/2 oz frozen sweetcorn
seasoning
Wholemeal shortcrust pastry
(see page 54)
semi-skimmed milk for brushing

Preheat the oven to 180°C/350°F/gas 4.

Heat the oil and soften the onion gently for 5 minutes. Add the garlic and mushrooms, cook for 1 minute and then sprinkle over the flour. Mix well. Remove from the heat and add the milk gradually, stirring well. Add the stock, return to the heat and bring the sauce to the boil. Simmer for 1 minute and then add the thyme, parsley, chicken, sweetcorn and seasoning. Transfer to a deep pie dish. Roll out the pastry and use to cover the pie. Brush with a little milk and bake for 40-45 minutes.

Opposite: Carrot and lentil soup *(top left*, see page 44); Lettuce soup *(top right*, see page 44); Hearty bean soup *(bottom*, see page 42)

Barbecued chicken with oven potatoes

Serves 4
Each serving: **260 kcal/1070 kJ, 20 g (2 exchanges) carbohydrate, 2 g fibre, 26 g protein, 7 g fat**

Oven potatoes
1 tbsp polyunsaturated
*   margarine*
1 tsp dried mixed herbs
400 g/14 oz potatoes, scrubbed
*   and cut into small pieces*
seasoning
3 tbsp water

Barbecue sauce
2 tbsp soy sauce
4 tbsp tomato purée
2 tbsp Worcester sauce
1 tsp dry mustard
6 tbsp water
1 tsp liquid sweetener
2 tbsp vinegar

4 portions chicken breast
*   (without skin)*
1 onion, chopped

Preheat the oven to 190°C/375°F/gas 5.

Melt the margarine with the herbs and toss the potato pieces in this. Transfer the potatoes to a casserole, season and add the water. Cover with a lid and cook in the oven for about 1 hour.

Lay the chicken portions in a flat ovenproof dish and sprinkle with the onion. Cook in the oven for 30 minutes. Make the Barbecue sauce by mixing the remaining ingredients together with a fork. Pour this over the chicken and bake for a further 30 minutes. (The potatoes and chicken should be ready to serve simultaneously.)

Sausage hot-pot

Serves 4
Each serving: 370 kcal/1550 kJ, 40 g (4 exchanges) carbohydrate, 5 g fibre, 21 g protein, 13 g fat

450 g/1 lb low-fat pork
*   sausagemeat*
1 medium-sized onion, finely
*   chopped*
1/2 tsp dried sage
1 small cooking apple, cored
*   and sliced*

400 g/14 oz canned tomatoes,
*   chopped with juice*
seasoning
500 g/11/4 lb potatoes,
*   scrubbed and thinly sliced*
25 g/3/4 oz Cheddar cheese,
*   grated*

Preheat the oven to 180°C/350°F/gas 4.

Spread the sausagemeat on the bottom of a casserole. Sprinkle over the chopped onion and sage. Arrange the apple slices on top. Pour over the tomatoes with the juice. Season well. Top this with the potato slices. Cover with a lid and bake for 1 hour; then remove the lid, sprinkle with the cheese and cook at 200°C/400°F/gas 6 for a further 30 minutes to brown the cheese.

Chilli con carne

Serves 4

Each serving: 250 kcal/1040 kJ, 20 g (2 exchanges) carbohydrate, 11 g fibre, 30 g protein, 5 g fat

150 g/5 oz red kidney beans,
  soaked in cold water overnight
400 g/14 oz lean minced beef
1 onion, chopped
1 green or red pepper, roughly chopped
1 clove garlic, crushed
1 tsp ground coriander

1 tsp ground cumin
1/2 tsp ground chilli
400 g/14 oz canned tomatoes,
  chopped with juice
300 ml/1/2 pint water
1 tsp dried mixed herbs
seasoning

Boil the beans hard for 10 minutes in fresh water and drain. Heat the minced beef in a large saucepan, slowly at first to release the fat, then turn up the heat and brown the meat well. Drain off any excess fat. Reduce the heat, add the onion, pepper and garlic, and cook gently for about 5 minutes before adding the spices. Cook for a further 1–2 minutes and then add the beans, tomatoes, water and herbs. Bring to the boil and simmer for 1 1/4 –1 1/2 hours until the beans are tender. (Alternatively, cook in a pressure cooker for 25 minutes.) Season to taste at the end of the cooking time and serve with bread or rice and salad.

Spicy lamb

Serves 4

Each serving: 360 kcal/1530 kJ, 20 g (2 exchanges) carbohydrate, 8 g fibre, 31 g protein, 18 g fat

150 g/5 oz dried butter beans, soaked
  in cold water for 6-8 hours
2 tbsp polyunsaturated oil
1 onion, chopped

1 clove garlic, crushed
450 g/1 lb lean lamb, cubed
2 tbsp tomato purée
1 tsp ground allspice
seasoning

Bring the beans to the boil in fresh water. Boil hard for 10 minutes, reduce the heat and simmer for about 30 minutes until they are almost tender.

Preheat the oven to 180°C/350°F/gas 4.

Heat 1 tbsp of the oil in a flameproof casserole and gently fry the onion for 5 minutes. Add the garlic and cook for a further 2 minutes. Remove the onion. Then brown the lamb in the remaining oil. Return the onion to the casserole with the tomato purée, allspice, butter beans and their liquid, and seasoning. Add enough water to just cover the meat. Cover with a lid and cook in the oven for about 1 hour or until tender.

Meat loaf

Serves 6

Each serving: 170 kcal/730 kJ, 10 g (1 exchange) carbohydrate, negligible fibre, 17 g protein, 8 g fat

1 1/2 tsp polyunsaturated oil
1 medium-sized onion, finely chopped

50 g/1 1/2 oz fresh wholemeal
  breadcrumbs

3 tbsp semi-skimmed milk
300 g/10¹/2 oz lean minced beef
200 g/7 oz low-fat sausagemeat
1 tbsp tomato purée

1 clove garlic, crushed
¹/2 tsp dried mixed herbs
seasoning
1 egg, beaten

Preheat the oven to 190°C/375°F/gas 5.

Heat the oil in a frying pan and soften the onion slowly without browning for about 5 minutes. Meanwhile, put the breadcrumbs and milk in a large bowl and leave to soak for 2–3 minutes. Then add the minced beef, sausagemeat, tomato purée, garlic, herbs, seasoning, the fried onion and beaten egg. Combine the ingredients until well mixed. (The easiest way to do this is with your hands.) Transfer the mixture to a 450 g/1 lb loaf tin, cover with foil and bake for 1 hour. Uncover and continue cooking for 30 minutes.

The meat loaf can be served hot or cold or used as a sandwich filling.

Cottage pie

Serves 4

Each serving: 290 kcal/1220 kJ, 40 g (4 exchanges) carbohydrate, 4 g fibre, 25 g protein, 5 g fat

Topping
600 g/1¹/2 lb potatoes, boiled
   and drained
2 tbsp natural yoghurt
seasoning

400 g/14 oz lean minced beef
1 large onion, finely chopped

¹/2 tsp thyme
¹/2 tsp basil
1 clove garlic, crushed
25 g/³/4 oz wholemeal flour
450 ml/³/4 pint beef stock
1 tsp tomato purée
seasoning

Mash the potatoes with the yoghurt and seasoning.

Heat the minced beef in a frying pan, slowly at first to release the fat, then turn up the heat and brown the meat well. Drain off any excess fat. Turn down the heat, add the onion and cook slowly until it becomes transparent. Add the herbs and garlic and sprinkle in the flour. Stir thoroughly, then add the stock gradually. Bring to the boil, stir in the tomato purée, season and simmer for 45 minutes.

Preheat the oven to 180°C/350°F/gas 4. Transfer the mixture to a deep pie dish, spread the mashed potato over the top and bake for 30 minutes.

Steak, kidney and bean pie

Serves 6

Each serving: 400 kcal/1693 kJ, 30 g (3 exchanges) carbohydrate, 6 g fibre, 23 g protein, 22 g fat

50 g/1¹/2 oz raw haricot beans,
   soaked in cold water overnight
1 tbsp polyunsaturated oil
350 g/12 oz lean chuck steak, cubed
175 g/6 oz kidney, cubed
2 medium-sized onions, chopped
450 ml/³/4 pint beef stock

1 tsp Worcester sauce
1 tsp dried mixed herbs
2 tsp tomato purée
seasoning

Wholemeal shortcrust pastry
200 g/7 oz wholemeal flour

50 g/1½ oz white vegetable fat
50 g/1½ oz polyunsaturated
  margarine

pinch salt
3 tbsp water
1 tsp polyunsaturated oil

Bring the beans to the boil in fresh water, boil hard for 10 minutes and drain. Heat the oil and brown the steak and kidney. Reduce the heat and add the onion. Cook gently for 3 minutes. Add the stock, flavourings, seasoning and drained beans to the pan. Bring to the boil and simmer for 1½ − 2 hours until the meat is tender and the beans just cooked. (Alternatively, pressure cook at high pressure for 25 minutes.)

Preheat the oven to 180°C/350°F/gas 4. Rub the fats into the flour and mix in the salt, then add the water and oil and work to a dough with a round-ended knife. Leave to stand for 10 minutes before rolling out. Transfer the cool meat mixture to a deep pie dish and season. Roll out the pastry and use to cover the pie dish. Bake for 40-45 minutes.

Spaghetti bolognese

Serves 6
Each serving: 360 kcal/1520 kJ, 40 g (4 exchanges) carbohydrate, 6 g fibre, 36 g protein, 9 g fat

650 g/1½ lb lean minced beef
200 g/7 oz chicken livers, finely
  chopped
2 medium-sized onions, finely
  chopped
1 clove garlic, crushed
400 g/14 oz canned tomatoes,
  chopped with juice

150 ml/¼ pint water
1 tsp dried oregano
seasoning

300 g/10½ oz wholemeal
  spaghetti
Parmesan cheese for sprinkling

Heat the minced beef in a saucepan, slowly at first to release the fat, then turn up the heat and brown the meat well. Drain off any excess fat. Add the chicken livers and onions and cook slowly for about 5 minutes, stirring from time to time. Add the garlic, tomatoes, water and oregano. Season well, cover with a lid and simmer gently for 40 minutes. Remove the lid and continue simmering for a further 30 minutes.

Cook the spaghetti in a large pan of boiling water for 10–15 minutes until just tender. Drain and serve with the meat sauce, sprinkling each portion lightly with Parmesan cheese.

Meaty macaroni bake

Serves 6
Each serving: 350 kcal/1470 kJ, 30 g (3 exchanges) carbohydrate, 5 g fibre, 27 g protein, 13 g fat

250 g/9 oz wholemeal macaroni
350 g/12 oz lean minced beef
1 onion, chopped
1 clove garlic, crushed
1 green pepper, chopped
½ tsp dried thyme

½ tsp dried oregano
2 eggs
450 ml/¾ pint semi-skimmed milk
seasoning
100 g/3½ oz Cheddar cheese, grated
3 tomatoes, sliced

Preheat the oven to 190°C/375°F/gas 5.

Boil the macaroni in plenty of water for 10–15 minutes until just tender.

Heat the minced beef in a saucepan, slowly at first to release the fat, then turn up the heat and brown the meat well. Drain off any excess fat. Add the onion, garlic and green pepper to the meat and cook gently for 5–10 minutes until the onion has softened. Add the herbs and mix well.

Drain the macaroni and mix with the mince, stirring well to combine them. Put the mixture into a shallow ovenproof dish. Whisk up the eggs with the milk and seasoning. Sprinkle the cheese over the macaroni, then arrange the tomato slices on top. Finally, pour over the egg and milk mixture and bake for 30–35 minutes until firm and just set.

Wholemeal pancakes

Makes 14

Each pancake: 60 kcal/250 kJ, 5 g (0.5 exchange) carbohydrate, negligible fibre, 2 g protein, 3 g fat

100 g/3¹/₂ oz wholemeal flour
2 eggs, beaten
200 ml/7 fl oz semi-skimmed milk

4 tbsp water
polyunsaturated oil for frying

Sift the flour into a bowl and make a well in the centre. Pour the eggs and a little milk into the well and gradually stir in the flour. Beat very hard to disperse any lumps before adding the remaining milk and water. Leave the batter to stand for 30 minutes.

Heat a little oil in a small heavy-based frying pan and when it is very hot, pour in 1¹/₂–2 tbsp of the batter. Swirl the pan to spread out the batter, then cook until it is firm and brown underneath. Turn with a palette knife or toss the pancake and cook the other side. Keep the pancakes warm on a plate in the oven while making the remainder. Serve with lemon juice and sugar-free sweetener or use as described in the following recipes for a main course.

Cooked pancakes can be frozen between layers of greaseproof paper.

Smoked fish pancakes

Serves 4

Each serving: 170 kcal/690 kJ, 10 g (1 exchange) carbohydrate, negligible fibre, 15 g protein, 9 g fat

Pancake batter (see above)
3 hard-boiled eggs, chopped
100 g/3¹/₂ oz cooked smoked
  haddock, flaked

4 tbsp skimmed milk soft cheese
pepper

Make the pancakes as described previously.

Preheat the oven to 200°C/400°F/gas 6.

Mix the hard-boiled eggs with the flaked fish and cheese, seasoning with pepper. Use this mixture to stuff the pancakes, rolling them up and arranging in a shallow ovenproof dish. Cover with foil and bake for 20 minutes. This dish can be prepared in advance and baked when required.

Cheese and ham pancakes

Serves 4
Each serving: 160 kcal/660 kJ, 10 g (1 exchange) carbohydrate, 1 g fibre, 19 g protein, 6 g fat

Pancake batter (see opposite)
350 g/12 oz cottage cheese
100 g/3¹/₂ oz lean ham, chopped

2 tbsp fresh chopped parsley
seasoning

Make the pancakes as described previously.
Preheat the oven to 200°C/400°F/gas 6.
Mix together the cottage cheese, ham, parsley and seasoning. Use this mixture to stuff the pancakes, rolling them up and arranging in a shallow ovenproof dish. Cover with foil and bake for 20 minutes. This dish can be prepared in advance and baked when required.

Pizza dough

Serves 4
Each serving: 220 kcal/910 kJ, 40 g (4 exchanges) carbohydrate, 6 g fibre, 10 g protein, 4 g fat

225 g/8 oz wholemeal flour
pinch of salt
2 tsp dried yeast
¹/₄ tsp fructose

100 ml/3¹/₂ fl oz warm water
1 egg, beaten
1 tsp polyunsaturated oil

Sift the flour and salt into a warm bowl. Stir the yeast and fructose into the warm water and leave in a warm place for 10 minutes or until frothy. Pour the egg and the yeast mixture into the flour and mix to a dough. Transfer the dough to a working surface and knead it for 10 minutes. Brush the surface of the dough with oil, cover and leave in a warm place until it has doubled in size (about 1 hour). Knead the dough again for 5 minutes, then roll it out to line a 30 cm/12 in diameter pizza tin or a Swiss roll tin (25 x 28 cm/10 x 11 in). Pinch up the edges to form a border. Cover the dough with the chosen topping.

Fishy pizza

Serves 4
Each serving: 300 kcal/1250 kJ, 40 g (4 exchanges) carbohydrate, 7 g fibre, 19 g protein, 8 g fat

Pizza dough (see above)
225 g/8 oz canned tomatoes, drained
1 tbsp tomato purée
¹/₂ tsp dried oregano
¹/₂ tsp dried basil

seasoning
125 g/4¹/₂ oz canned sardines
 in oil, drained and mashed
2 tbsp cottage cheese
3-4 stuffed olives, sliced

Roll out the pizza dough to the desired shape. Rub the tomatoes through a sieve using a wooden spoon. Stir the tomato puree, herbs and seasoning into the tomato pulp. Spread this mixture over the prepared pizza dough. Arrange the sardines, cottage cheese and olives on top of the sauce. Leave the pizza to rise a little for 10 minutes.

Preheat the oven to 220°C/425°F/gas 7. Bake the pizza for 15–20 minutes.

Bacon and mushroom pizza See photograph, page 60

Serves 4

Each serving: 280 kcal/1170 kJ, 40 g (4 exchanges) carbohydrate, 7 g fibre, 18 g protein, 7 g fat

Pizza dough (see page 57)
225 g/8 oz canned tomatoes, drained
1 tbsp tomato purée
1/2 tsp dried oregano
1/2 tsp dried thyme

seasoning
100 g/3 1/2 oz lean bacon, chopped
50 g/1 1/2 oz mushrooms, sliced
25 g/3/4 oz cheese, grated

Roll out the pizza dough to the desired shape. Rub the tomatoes through a sieve using a wooden spoon. Stir the tomato purée, herbs and seasoning into the tomato pulp. Spread this mixture on top of the pizza dough. Scatter the bacon, mushrooms and cheese over the top and leave the pizza to rise a little for 10–15 minutes.

Preheat the oven to 220°C/425°F/gas 7. Bake the pizza for 15–20 minutes.

Pancakes bolognese See photograph, page 60

Serves 4

Each serving: 290 kcal/1230 kJ, 10 g (1 exchange) carbohydrate, 1 g fibre, 29 g protein, 16 g fat

Pancake batter (see page 56)
1/2 quantity of Bolognese sauce
(see page 55)

75 g/2 1/2 oz Cheddar cheese,
grated

Make the pancakes as described previously.

Preheat the oven to 200°C/400°F/gas 6.

Put a little of the Bolognese sauce on each pancake, roll up and lay in a shallow ovenproof dish. Sprinkle with the grated cheese and bake for 20 minutes. This dish can be prepared in advance and baked when required.

Opposite: Green 'crunch' salad (*top*, see page 45); Rainbow salad (*centre*, see page 45); Red cabbage and pineapple salad (*bottom*, see page 45)
Overleaf: Pancakes bolognese (*left*); Tuna spaghetti (*centre*, see page 47); Bacon and mushroom pizza (*right and bottom*)

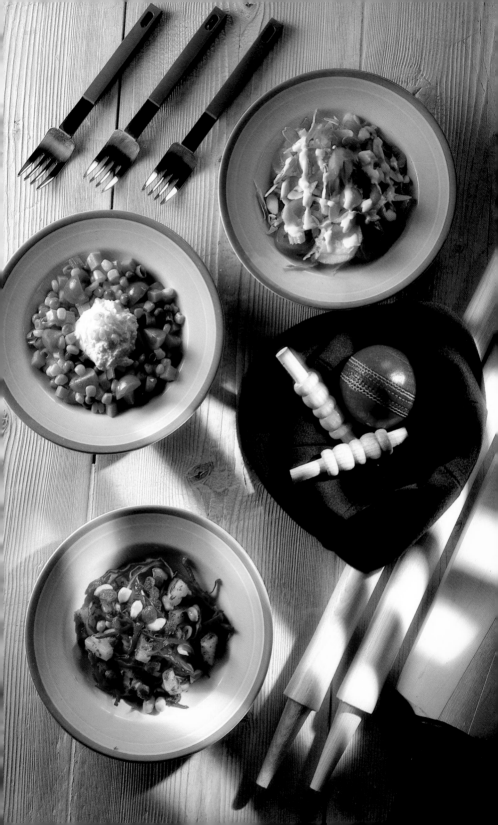

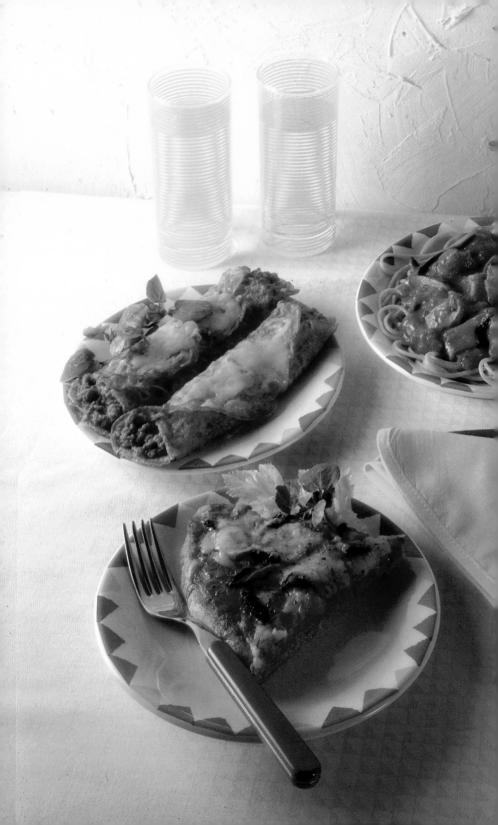

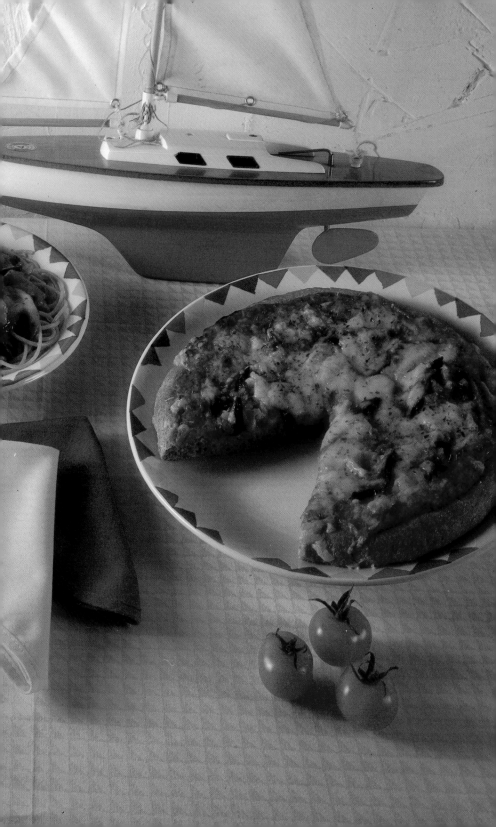

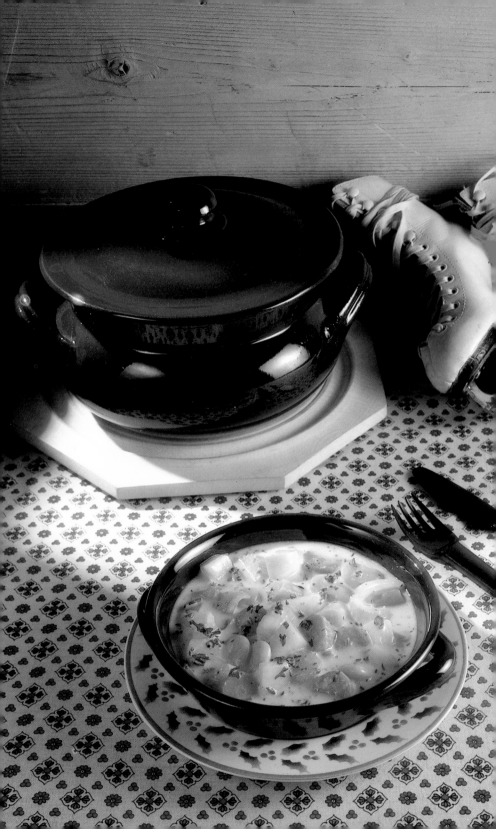

VEGETARIAN DISHES

Creamy winter stew

Serves 4

Each serving: 290 kcal/1210 kJ, 40 g (4 exchanges) carbohydrate, 18 g fibre, 18 g protein, 6 g fat

200 g/7 oz dried butter beans,
*   soaked in cold water for 6–8 hours*
1 tbsp polyunsaturated oil
1 onion, chopped
3 leeks, cut into 2.5 cm/1 in chunks
2 carrots, diced
2 celery stalks, cut into 2.5 cm/
*   1 in pieces*

375 ml/³/₄ pint semi-skimmed milk
handful of chopped parsley
1 tsp dried thyme
2 tsp yeast extract
seasoning
150 g/5 oz potato, diced

Bring the beans to the boil in fresh water, boil hard for 10 minutes then simmer for 20 minutes. Heat the oil in a large pan and soften the onion by cooking slowly for 3–5 minutes. Add the leeks, carrots and celery. Cover with a lid and sweat the vegetables for 10 minutes, stirring occasionally to prevent browning. Add the milk, parsley, thyme and yeast extract. Season well. Add the drained beans and simmer for 20 minutes before adding the potato. Simmer for a further 30–40 minutes until the vegetables and beans are cooked and the sauce has thickened. Adjust the seasoning to taste. The stew can be frozen.

Nut loaf

Serves 6

Each serving: 260 kcal/1090 kJ, 20 g (2 exchanges) carbohydrate, 3 g fibre, 7 g protein, 19 g fat

50 g/1¹/₂ oz polyunsaturated
*   margarine*
1 onion, finely chopped
100 g/3¹/₂ oz mushrooms, chopped
1 egg
300 ml/¹/₂ pint semi-skimmed milk

100 g/3¹/₂ oz nuts (mixed hazelnuts,
*   Brazil nuts, walnuts and almonds),*
*   finely chopped*
100 g/3¹/₂ oz rolled oats
¹/₂ tsp dried mixed herbs
seasoning

Lightly oil and line with greaseproof paper the base of a 450 g/1 lb loaf tin. Preheat the oven to 180°C/350°F/gas 4.

Melt the margarine and cook the onion gently for 5 minutes. Add the mushrooms and cook for a further 2–3 minutes. Beat the egg with the milk. Mix together the nuts, oats and herbs, add the onion and mushrooms with the egg mixture. Season well and mix together thoroughly. Turn into the loaf tin and bake for 1 hour until firm. Serve hot or cold, cut into slices. If serving hot, leave to cool in the tin for 1–2 minutes before turning out and slicing.

Opposite: Creamy winter stew

Glamorgan sausages

Makes 8

Each sausage: 170 kcal/700 kJ, 10 g (1 exchange) carbohydrate, 2 g fibre, 8 g protein, 11 g fat

125 g/4¹/₂ oz Cheddar cheese, grated
100 g/3¹/₂ oz fresh wholemeal
  breadcrumbs
2 tbsp very finely chopped leek
1 egg
1 egg yolk
¹/₂ tsp dried thyme
1 tsp dry mustard
seasoning
polyunsaturated oil for frying

To coat
1 egg white
75 g/2¹/₂ oz fresh wholemeal
  breadcrumbs

Mix together the cheese, breadcrumbs and leek. Whisk the whole egg, the egg yolk, herb, mustard and seasoning. Pour this into the cheese mixture and combine together. Divide the mixture into eight equal portions and roll into small sausages.

Break up the egg white with a fork on a plate and roll the sausages in this. Coat each with the breadcrumbs, chill for 15–20 minutes and fry until golden in a small amount of hot oil. This will take about 5–7 minutes.

Leek lasagne

Serves 4

Each serving: 270 kcal/1130 kJ, 30 g (3 exchanges) carbohydrate, 5 g fibre, 12 g protein, 13 g fat

Leek sauce
2 medium leeks, chopped
1 tbsp polyunsaturated oil
50 g/1¹/₂ oz mushrooms, sliced
400 g/14 oz canned tomatoes,
  chopped with juice
1 clove garlic
¹/₂ tsp dried thyme
seasoning

Cheese sauce
300 ml/¹/₂ pint semi-skimmed
  milk
15 g/¹/₂ oz polyunsaturated
  margarine
15 g/¹/₂ oz plain flour
50 g/1¹/₂ oz mature Cheddar
  cheese, grated
seasoning

100 g/3¹/₂ oz wholemeal lasagne

Prepare the Leek sauce by softening the leeks in the oil over a low heat for a few minutes, then adding all the other ingredients and simmering for 20 minutes.

Preheat the oven to 180°C/350°F/gas 4.

Prepare the Cheese sauce by whisking the milk, margarine and flour continuously over the heat. When the sauce has boiled and thickened, remove from the heat, stir in the grated cheese and season. Layer the uncooked lasagne with the two sauces in a shallow ovenproof dish ending with a layer of cheese sauce. Bake the lasagne for 1 hour.

Cabbage macaroni gratin

Serves 4
Each serving: 330 kcal/1380 kJ, 40 g (4 exchanges) carbohydrate, 5 g fibre, 15 g protein, 15 g fat

100 g/3¹/₂ oz wholemeal macaroni
200 g/7 oz shredded white cabbage
450 ml/³/₄ pint semi-skimmed
  milk
25 g/³/₄ oz polyunsaturated
  margarine
50 g/1¹/₂ oz wholemeal flour

75 g/2¹/₂ oz mature Cheddar
  cheese, grated
seasoning
¹/₂ tsp dry mustard
25 g/³/₄ oz fresh wholemeal
  breadcrumbs

Preheat the oven to 180°C/350°F/gas 4.

Cook the macaroni in a large pan of fast-boiling water for 7 minutes. Add the shredded cabbage to the macaroni, bring back to the boil and boil for 3 minutes.

Meanwhile make a sauce by whisking together the milk, margarine and flour over the heat until it boils and thickens. Simmer for 1 minute. Add the cheese, reserving a little for the topping, season and add the mustard.

Drain the macaroni and cabbage and put in a flat ovenproof dish. Pour over the sauce. Sprinkle the breadcrumbs and reserved cheese over the top and bake for 15–20 minutes.

Vegetable crumble

Serves 6
Each serving: 220 kcal/940 kJ, 30 g (3 exchanges) carbohydrate, 10 g fibre, 9 g protein, 7 g fat

125 g/4¹/₂ oz haricot beans, soaked
  in cold water for 6–8 hours
1 tbsp polyunsaturated oil
1 onion, finely chopped
1 carrot, diced
1 celery stalk, diced
50 g/1¹/₂ oz mushrooms, sliced
2 potatoes, diced
2 courgettes or equivalent
  quantity of marrow, sliced

1 tsp dried mixed herbs
1 tbsp tomato purée
400 g/14 oz canned tomatoes,
  chopped with juice

Topping
25 g/³/₄ oz polyunsaturated
  margarine
50 g/1¹/₂ oz fresh wholemeal
  breadcrumbs
50 g/1¹/₂ oz rolled oats

Bring the beans to the boil in fresh water, boil hard for 10 minutes then simmer until tender.

Heat the oil in a saucepan and cook the onion, carrot and celery gently until they soften a little. Add the mushrooms, potatoes, courgettes, herbs, tomato purée and tomatoes. Season well, bring to the boil and simmer for 20 minutes. Mix in the beans and transfer to an ovenproof pie dish.

Preheat the oven to 180°C/350°F/gas 4. Mix the topping ingredients together with a fork until the margarine is well dispersed. Spread this mixture on top of the vegetables and bake for 25–30 minutes.

Bulghur wheat pilaff

Serves 6

Each serving: 220 kcal/930 kJ, 30 g (3 exchanges) carbohydrate, 3 g fibre, 7 g protein, 8 g fat

200 g/7 oz bulghur (cracked wheat)
600 ml/1 pint vegetable stock
1 tbsp polyunsaturated oil
1 onion, chopped
1 red pepper, chopped
50 g/1½ oz toasted hazelnuts

25 g/¾ oz sunflower seeds
100 g/3½ oz cooked continental lentils
100 g/3½ oz mushrooms, sliced
seasoning

Put the bulghur and stock into a large pan and bring to the boil. Simmer gently for about 10 minutes until the bulghur has swollen and absorbed the stock.

Heat the oil in a large frying pan or wok and soften the chopped onion and red pepper slowly. Add the cooked bulghur together with all the remaining ingredients. Heat gently, stirring all the time, until well heated through. Season to taste and serve immediately.

Lentil burgers

Makes 10

Each burger: 120 kcal/520 kJ, 10 g (1 exchange) carbohydrate, 3 g fibre, 6 g protein, 5 g fat

200 g/7 oz red lentils
25 g/¾ oz polyunsaturated margarine
½ onion, grated
1 tsp ground coriander
1 tsp yeast extract

1 tbsp chopped parsley
pepper
50 g/1½ oz wholemeal flour for coating
polyunsaturated oil for frying

Cover the lentils with cold water and simmer until tender – about 30 minutes. Drain and mash the lentils.

Melt the margarine and soften the grated onion in it for 2–3 minutes. Add the coriander and cook for a further minute. Mix the onion, yeast extract, parsley and pepper with the lentils and cool. Shape into ten burgers with wet hands and coat each one in a little flour. Chill for 5–10 minutes. Fry in a little oil for 5 minutes on each side. The burgers may be frozen before cooking. Open freeze and transfer to an airtight container when frozen.

Nut balls

Makes 10

Each nut ball: 130 kcal/550 kJ, 5 g (0.5 exchange) carbohydrate, 3 g fibre, 5 g protein, 10 g fat

1 onion, finely chopped
1 tbsp polyunsaturated oil
175 g/6 oz ground mixed nuts (not peanuts)
25 g/¾ oz soya flour

75 g/2½ oz fresh wholemeal breadcrumbs
1 tsp dried mixed herbs
seasoning
1 egg, beaten

Preheat the oven to 200°C/400°F/gas 6.

Fry the onion in the oil very gently to soften but not brown it. Leave to cool a little. Mix together the nuts, soya flour, breadcrumbs, herbs and seasoning in a bowl. Add the beaten egg and onion, mixing well. Form the mixture into ten equal-sized balls, using wet hands. Chill for 5–10 minutes then bake for 20 minutes and serve with Tomato sauce (see page 69) or Ratatouille sauce (see page 68). The nut balls may be frozen before cooking. Open freeze and transfer to an airtight container when frozen.

Spaghetti and courgette cheese

Serves 4

Each serving: 270 kcal/1150 kJ, 40 g (4 exchanges) carbohydrate, 6 g fibre, 11 g protein, 10 g fat

200 g/7 oz wholemeal spaghetti
300 g/10¹/₂ oz courgettes, cut into
* 1 cm/¹/₂ in slices*
25 g/³/₄ oz polyunsaturated margarine

seasoning
1 clove garlic, crushed
50 g/1¹/₂ oz Parmesan or other
* hard cheese, grated*

Put the spaghetti into a large pan of fast-boiling water and boil for 10 minutes. Add the courgettes to the pan and cook for a further 5 minutes. Tip the pasta and courgettes into a colander.

Melt the margarine in the saucepan and add the seasoning and garlic. When the fat is sizzling, return the spaghetti and courgettes to the pan. Toss well and serve immediately, sprinkled with the cheese.

Courgette rice bake

Serves 6

Each serving: 260 kcal/1070 kJ, 40 g (4 exchanges) carbohydrate, 3 g fibre, 8 g protein, 9 g fat

1 tbsp polyunsaturated oil
1 onion, chopped
200 g/7 oz brown rice
1 tsp mixed dried herbs
600 ml/1 pint vegetable stock
375 ml/³/₄ pint semi-skimmed milk
25 g/³/₄ oz polyunsaturated margarine
25 g/³/₄ oz wholemeal flour

25 g/³/₄ oz mature Cheddar cheese,
* grated*
¹/₂ tsp dry mustard
seasoning
4 tomatoes, sliced
¹/₂ tsp dried basil
300 g/10¹/₂ oz courgettes, sliced

Heat the oil in a saucepan and cook the onion gently for 2–3 minutes. Add the rice and stir well until coated with oil. Add the herbs and stock, bring to the boil and simmer gently for 40–45 minutes until the rice is tender and the stock absorbed.

Meanwhile make a cheese sauce by whisking the milk, margarine and flour together over the heat until boiling and thickened. Stir in the cheese, mustard and seasoning.

Preheat the oven to 160°C/325°F/gas 4.

Transfer the cooked rice to a shallow ovenproof dish. Arrange the sliced tomatoes on this and sprinkle with the basil. Put the sliced courgettes on top, then pour over the cheese sauce. Bake for 30–35 minutes until the top is golden and the courgettes are just cooked.

Cheese and vegetable pizza

Serves 4

Each serving: 340 kcal/1440 kJ, 40 g (4 exchanges) carbohydrate, 8 g fibre, 17 g protein, 13 g fat

Pizza dough (see page 57)
1 tbsp polyunsaturated oil
1 onion, finely chopped
1 celery stalk, finely chopped
¹/₂ green pepper, finely chopped

400 g/14 oz canned tomatoes,
  chopped with juice
1 tbsp tomato purée
1 tsp mixed dried herbs
seasoning
75 g/2¹/₂ oz Cheddar cheese, grated

Roll out the pizza dough to the desired shape (about 1 cm/¹/₂ in thick).

Heat the oil and cook the onion, celery and green pepper gently for 5–10 minutes until slightly softened but not brown. Add the tomatoes, tomato purée, mixed herbs and seasoning. Bring to the boil and simmer for 20–30 minutes. Purée the vegetables in a blender, food processor or by rubbing through a sieve. Spread this purée thickly over the pizza dough. Sprinkle with the grated cheese and leave the pizza to rise a little for about 10 minutes.

Preheat the oven to 220°C/425°F/gas 7 and bake the pizza for 15–20 minutes.

Ratatouille sauce

Serves 4

Each serving: 100 kcal/420 kJ, 10 g (1 exchange) carbohydrate, 3 g fibre, 2 g protein, 8 g fat

1 aubergine, diced
pinch salt
2 tbsp polyunsaturated oil
1 onion, chopped
1 green pepper, chopped
2 courgettes, sliced

400 g/14 oz canned tomatoes,
  chopped with juice
2 tbsp tomato purée
2 tsp dried basil
black pepper

Layer the diced aubergine in a colander, sprinkling each layer with a little salt. Cover with a plate, held down with a weight, and leave for 30-40 minutes to drain off the bitter juices. Rinse and dry the aubergine on kitchen paper.

Heat the oil in a large saucepan and cook the onion and pepper together for about 5 minutes. Add the diced aubergine and sliced courgettes and continue cooking over a moderate heat for 5–7 minutes, stirring occasionally. Add the tomatoes, tomato purée and basil. Season well with black pepper, cover and cook gently for 30 minutes. Purée or liquidize the vegetables to a sauce and adjust the seasoning to taste before serving.

Tomato sauce

Serves 4
Each serving: 50 kcal/210 kJ, 5 g (0.5 exchange) carbohydrate, 1 g fibre, 2 g protein, 3 g fat

1 tbsp polyunsaturated oil
1 onion, finely chopped
1 clove garlic, crushed
400 g/14 oz canned tomatoes,
   chopped with juice

1 tbsp tomato purée
1 tsp dried oregano or basil
seasoning

Heat the oil and fry the onion slowly for 5 minutes until it looks transparent. Add the garlic, tomatoes and juice, tomato purée and oregano or basil. Season well and simmer, covered, for 15 minutes. Remove the lid and continue cooking gently for a further 10–15 minutes until the sauce thickens. The sauce may be sieved or liquidized if a smooth result is preferred. Serve with fish cakes, nut balls, lentil burgers, for example.

Leek flan   See photograph, page 71

Serves 6
Each serving: 260 kcal/1080 kJ, 20 g (2 exchanges) carbohydrate, 4 g fibre, 8 g protein, 17 g fat

Nut pastry
25 g/³/4 oz white vegetable fat
25 g/³/4 oz polyunsaturated margarine
100 g/3¹/2 oz wholemeal flour
50 g/1¹/2 oz ground hazelnuts
2–3 tbsp water

Filling
25 g/³/4 oz polyunsaturated margarine
300 g/10¹/2 oz leeks, finely chopped
25 g/³/4 oz wholemeal flour
300 ml/¹/2 pint semi-skimmed milk
1 egg, beaten
3 tbsp skimmed milk soft cheese
seasoning

Rub the fats into the flour. Stir in the ground hazelnuts. Mix in enough water with a round-ended knife to form a dough. Leave to stand for 10 minutes.

Melt the margarine in a saucepan, add the chopped leek, cover and cook gently for 5 minutes. Add the flour and cook, stirring, for 2 minutes. Remove from the heat and add the milk gradually, stirring well. Return to the heat, bring to the boil and simmer for 2–3 minutes, stirring constantly. Cool the leek mixture. (For a smoother result the filling may be liquidized at this stage.)

Preheat the oven to 190°C/375°F/gas 5. Roll out the pastry to line a 20 cm /8 in flan ring. Beat the egg and soft cheese into the leek sauce, season and pour into the pastry case. Bake for 35–40 minutes until set.

Three-bean risotto See photograph, page 71

Serves 4

Each serving: 300 kcal/1240 kJ, 50 g (5 exchanges) carbohydrate, 5 g fibre, 12 g protein, 6 g fat

1 tbsp polyunsaturated oil
1 onion, chopped
200 g/7 oz brown rice
600 ml/1 pint vegetable stock
400 g/14 oz canned tomatoes,
  chopped with juice
1/2 tsp dried oregano

seasoning
1 medium-sized red pepper, diced
100 g/3¹/₂ oz cooked red kidney beans
100 g/3¹/₂ oz frozen or fresh cut
  green beans
100 g/3¹/₂ oz bean sprouts
100 g/3¹/₂ oz cottage cheese

Heat the oil in a large frying pan or wok. Add the onion and cook slowly for 5 minutes. Add the rice and continue cooking for 2–3 minutes, stirring continuously. Add the stock, tomatoes, oregano and seasoning. Cover and simmer for 35–40 minutes until rice is almost tender. Add the red pepper, kidney beans, green beans and bean sprouts and simmer for a further 5 minutes. Add the cottage cheese, mix together thoroughly and serve immediately.

Opposite: Three-bean risotto (*top*); Leek flan (*bottom*, see page 69)

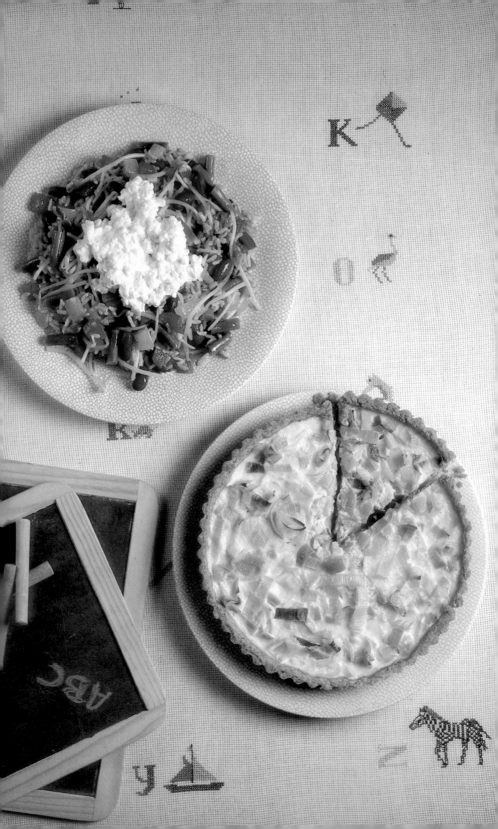

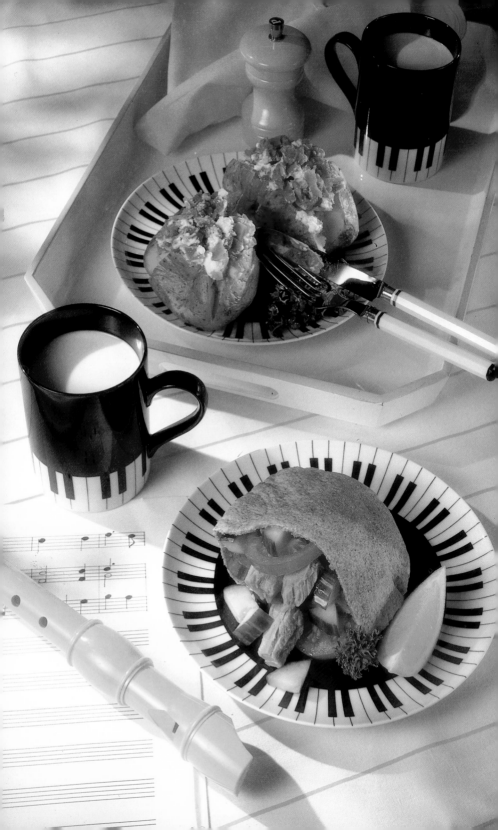

SNACKS AND LIGHT MEALS

Pitta bread with tuna

Serves 4
Each serving: 200 kcal/860 kJ, 30 g (3 exchanges) carbohydrate, 4 g fibre, 19 g protein, 1 g fat

2 wholemeal pitta breads
200 g/7 oz canned tuna fish in
* brine, drained*
1/2 cucumber, diced

2 tomatoes, diced
2 tbsp lemon juice
black pepper

Put the pitta breads under a hot grill and cook until they expand, turning once. Mix together the tuna, cucumber, tomato and lemon juice, seasoning well with freshly ground black pepper.

Cut the pittas in half width-ways, and fill each half with a quarter of the tuna mixture. Serve immediately.

Ham and peanut potatoes

Serves 4
Each serving: 260 kcal/1092 kJ, 40 g (4 exchanges) carbohydrate, 4 g fibre, 15 g protein, 6 g fat

4 potatoes, each 175 g/6 oz
100 g/31/2 oz lean cooked ham,
* finely chopped*

2 tbsp crunchy peanut butter
4 tbsp skimmed milk soft cheese
seasoning

Preheat the oven to 180°C/350°F/gas 4.

Scrub the potatoes thoroughly and dry them. Bake for 1 1/2 –2 hours or until potatoes are soft.

Mix the ham with the peanut butter and soft cheese, and season. Split open the cooked potatoes and divide the filling between them.

Cheese and pickle potatoes

Serves 4
Each serving: 260 kcal/1092 kJ, 40 g (4 exchanges) carbohydrate, 4 g fibre, 10 g protein, 9 g fat

4 potatoes, each 175 g/6 oz
100 g/31/2 oz Cheddar cheese, grated

2 tbsp pickle

Preheat the oven to 180°C/350°F/gas 4.

Bake the potatoes as described above.

Opposite: Ham and peanut potatoes(*top*); Pitta bread with tuna (*bottom*)

Mix together the cheese and pickle, blending well with a fork. Divide the mixture equally between the potatoes.

Onion hot dogs

Serves 4
Each serving: 260 kcal/1090 kJ, 30 g (3 exchanges) carbohydrate, 5 g fibre, 13 g protein, 11 g fat

4 large low-fat pork sausages
1 tbsp polyunsaturated oil
1 medium-sized onion, finely sliced
1 tbsp soy sauce

2 tbsp tomato purée
2 tbsp water
4 wholemeal rolls

Grill the sausages for 20 minutes, turning as required. While they cook, heat the oil in a saucepan and add the onion. Cook fairly briskly until golden and softened. Add the soy sauce, tomato purée and water and mix well over the heat.

Split the rolls, divide the onion mixture between them and place a sausage in each.

Sweetcorn fritters

Makes 8
Each fritter: 80 kcal/350 kJ, 10 g (1 exchange) carbohydrate, 2 g fibre, 3 g protein, 5 g fat

50 g/1¹/₂ oz wholemeal flour
1 egg
2 tbsp semi-skimmed milk

200 g/7 oz canned sweetcorn, drained
seasoning
polyunsaturated oil for frying

Put the flour in a bowl, make a well in the centre and break the egg into it. Add the milk and, with a hand whisk or wooden spoon, mix the flour into the egg and milk gradually. Beat the mixture well. Add the sweetcorn and season.

Heat a little oil in a frying pan. Add tablespoonfuls of the batter to form fritters. Allow the mixture to become firm and brown before turning once to cook on the other side, about 2–3 minutes per side.

Quick bacon stir-fry

Serves 4
Each serving: 230 kcal/970 kJ, 40 g (4 exchanges) carbohydrate, 3 g fibre, 12 g protein, 4 g fat

150 g/5 oz lean bacon, chopped
50 g/1¹/₂ oz frozen peas
500 g/1¹/₄ lb cooked brown rice

50 g/1¹/₂ oz frozen sweetcorn
2 tomatoes, chopped
seasoning

Cook the bacon in its own fat in a large frying pan until it begins to crisp. Add the (uncooked) peas and sweetcorn to the pan and fry briskly, stirring continuously, for 3–4 minutes. Add the rice and continue stir-frying until the rice is heated through. Finally add the chopped tomatoes and seasoning. Cook for a further 2 minutes and then serve immediately.

Beef and liver burgers

Makes 6
Each burger: 140 kcal/580 kJ, 5 g (0.5 exchange) carbohydrate, negligible fibre, 17 g protein, 6 g fat

350 g/12 oz lean minced beef
100 g/3½ oz lamb's liver
4 tbsp fresh wholemeal breadcrumbs
1 tsp dried mixed herbs

1 tbsp soy sauce
1 tbsp Worcester sauce
1 egg
polyunsaturated oil for frying

Mince the beef and liver together and combine the meat with all the other ingredients. Form the mixture into six burgers using wet hands. Fry in a little polyunsaturated oil or grill for 7 minutes on each side.

Rice fritters

Makes 10
Each fritter: 110 kcal/440 kJ, 10 g (1 exchange) carbohydrate, negligible fibre, 3 g protein, 7 g fat

150 g/5 oz cooked brown rice
50 g/1½ oz Cheddar cheese, grated
1 small onion, grated
25 g/¾ oz self-raising wholemeal
* flour*

2 tbsp semi-skimmed milk
1 egg, beaten
½ tsp yeast extract
pepper
polyunsaturated oil for frying

Beat all the ingredients together in a bowl. Heat a little oil in a frying pan and put tablespoonfuls of the mixture into it to make fritters. Fry briskly for 3–4 minutes and when the fritters are firm and brown underneath, turn them to cook on the other side. Keep them hot in the oven while the remaining mixture is cooked.

PACKED LUNCHES

Sandwiches

The quantities given in the following fillings are sufficient to make two rounds of sandwiches (that is, four slices of wholemeal bread taken from a large pre-sliced loaf). The nutritional analyses, however, apply to one sandwich only (that is, two slices of wholemeal bread).

It is recommended that the bread is spread very thinly with polyunsaturated margarine before making the sandwiches.

Ham and soft cheese filling

Each sandwich: 230 kcal/970 kJ, 30 g (3 exchanges) carbohydrate, 5 g fibre, 12 g protein, 10 g fat

*50 g/1½ oz lean ham, finely
   chopped*

*2 tbsp skimmed milk soft cheese
½ tsp French mustard*

Mix all the ingredients together.

Carrot and cheese filling See photograph, page 81

Each sandwich: 260 kcal/1080 kJ, 30 g (3 exchanges) carbohydrate, 6 g fibre, 10 g protein, 13 g fat

*30 g/1 oz carrot, grated
30 g/1 oz Cheddar cheese, grated*

*1 tbsp natural yoghurt
seasoning*

Mix all the ingredients together.

Egg and celery filling

Each sandwich: 280 kcal/1190 kJ, 30 g (3 exchanges) carbohydrate, 5 g fibre, 9 g protein, 17 g fat

*1 hard-boiled egg, chopped
1 celery stalk, finely chopped*

*1 tbsp mayonnaise
seasoning*

Mix all the ingredients together.

Banana and peanut butter filling

Each sandwich: 250 kcal/1060 kJ, 30 g (3 exchanges) carbohydrate, 6 g fibre, 7 g protein, 12 g fat

*½ banana, mashed with 1 tsp lemon
   juice*

1 tbsp peanut butter

Spread the peanut butter on the bread and top with mashed banana.

Cottage cheese and apricot filling See photograph, page 81

Each sandwich: 210 kcal/860 kJ, 30 g (3 exchanges) carbohydrate, 5 g fibre, 7 g protein, 9 g fat

2 tbsp cottage cheese, sieved
2 tbsp apricot purée

sugar-free sweetener to taste

Mix the cottage cheese with the apricot purée and sweeten to taste.

Liver sausage and pickle filling See photograph, page 81

Each sandwich: 280 kcal/1160 kJ, 30 g (3 exchanges) carbohydrate, 5 g fibre, 9 g protein, 15 g fat

50 g/1¹/₂ oz liver sausage, sliced   *1 tbsp pickle*

Arrange the sliced liver sausage on the bread and spread the pickle on top.

Cheese and strawberry filling

Each sandwich: 210 kcal/890 kJ, 30 g (3 exchanges) carbohydrate, 5 g fibre, 7 g protein, 9 g fat

2 tbsp skimmed milk soft cheese   *2 tsp low-sugar strawberry jam*

Spread the cheese on to the bread, followed by a thin spreading of the jam.

Sausage and tomato filling

Each sandwich: 300 kcal/1280 kJ, 30 g (3 exchanges) carbohydrate, 6 g fibre, 10 g protein, 17 g fat

1 large, cold cooked sausage, diced   *1 tbsp mayonnaise*
1 large tomato, diced   *1 tsp tomato ketchup*

Bind the diced sausage and tomato with the mayonnaise and ketchup.

For other fillings, see Smoked mackerel pâté (below), Sardine pâté (page 78), Spicy split pea pâté (page 78) and Meat loaf (page 53).

Smoked mackerel pâté

Serves 6
Each serving: 150 kcal/630 kJ, negligible carbohydrate, negligible fibre, 14 g protein, 10 g fat

2 medium-sized smoked
*   mackerel fillets*
100 g/3¹/₂ oz cottage cheese

75 ml/2¹/₂ fl oz natural yoghurt
juice of 1/2 lemon
2 tsp horseradish sauce

Remove the skin and any bones from the mackerel fillets. Mix the fish with all the other ingredients in a liquidizer or food processor until smooth and creamy. Use as a pâté or sandwich filling.

Sardine pâté

Serves 6

Each serving: 110 kcal/470 kJ, 5 g (0.5 exchange) carbohydrate, negligible fibre, 11 g protein, 6 g fat

2 x 125 g/4¹/₂ oz cans sardines in oil
50 g/1¹/₂ oz fresh wholemeal
*   breadcrumbs*
grated rind and juice of 1 lemon

2 tbsp natural yoghurt
2 tbsp chopped parsley
seasoning

Drain the oil from the sardines, reserving 1 tbsp. Mash the sardines and the reserved oil with a fork, then mix in the other ingredients. Blend thoroughly until a fairly smooth consistency is achieved.

Spicy split pea pâté

Serves 4

Each serving: 230 kcal/950 kJ, 30 g (3 exchanges) carbohydrate, 6 g fibre, 11 g protein, 8 g fat

200 g/7 oz yellow split peas
¹/₂ small onion, grated
¹/₂ fresh green chilli (optional), finely
*   chopped*

1 small clove garlic, crushed
juice of ¹/₂ lemon
2 tbsp polyunsaturated oil
paprika (to garnish)

Cover the peas with cold water in a saucepan, cover with a lid and bring to the boil. Simmer very gently for 30 minutes until the peas are soft and have absorbed the water. Mash the peas with all the other ingredients. Sprinkle with paprika immediately before serving cold with salads. This pâté freezes well.

Crunchy drumsticks

Serves 4

Each serving: 140 kcal/590 kJ, 5 g (0.5 exchange) carbohydrate, negligible fibre, 16 g protein, 6 g fat

25 g/³/₄ oz toasted wheatflakes
25 g/³/₄ oz Cheddar cheese, grated

pinch each dried thyme, sage
*   and rosemary*
4 chicken drumsticks
*   (without skin)*

Preheat the oven to 160°C/325°F/gas 3.

Mix the wheatflakes with the cheese and herbs and press this mixture on to the drumsticks to coat them. Bake for 30–40 minutes until the chicken is cooked through. Serve cold.

Savoury slice

Makes 20 slices

Each slice: 120 kcal/490 kJ, 10 g (1 exchange) carbohydrate, 1 g fibre, 5 g protein, 7 g fat

250 g/9 oz jumbo oats

1 onion, grated

2 carrots, grated
1 celery stalk, grated or finely chopped
200 g/7 oz Cheddar cheese, grated
1 tsp mixed dried herbs

50 g/1½ oz polyunsaturated margarine
1 egg, beaten
seasoning

Preheat the oven to 180°C/350°F/gas 4.

Mix together the oats, grated vegetables, cheese and herbs. Melt the margarine; add to the oat mixture with the beaten egg. Season well and mix thoroughly. Spread the mixture into a Swiss roll tin, and bake for 25–30 minutes until firm and golden. Cut into twenty slices while still hot but leave to cool in the tin.

Sausage apple plait

Makes 8 slices
Each slice: 170 kcal/700 kJ, 10 g (1 exchange) carbohydrate, 2 g fibre, 6 g protein, 10 g fat

225 g/8 oz low-fat sausagemeat
50 g/1½ oz leek, finely chopped
50 g/1½ oz cooking apple, grated
1 tsp dried sage

seasoning
Wholemeal shortcrust pastry
  (see page 54)
semi-skimmed milk for brushing

Preheat the oven to 190°C/375°F/gas 5.

Mix the sausagemeat with the leek, apple and sage, and season. Form the mixture into a 'sausage' about 25 cm/10 in long. Roll out the pastry to a rectangle about 25 x 23 cm/10 x 9 in. Lay the 'sausage' down the centre of the pastry. Make slits with a knife about 2.5 cm/1 in apart down each side of the pastry. Brush with water, then fold over pieces of the pastry from alternate sides to make a 'plait'. Transfer to a baking tray. Brush with milk, then bake for 1–1¼ hours. Allow to cool before removing from the baking sheet. Cut into eight slices.

Bean and pepper flan

Serves 4
Each serving: 530 kcal/2217 kJ, 30 g (3 exchanges) carbohydrate, 7 g fibre, 17 g protein, 37 g fat

Pastry
40 g/1⅓ oz polyunsaturated
  margarine
35 g/1¼ oz white vegetable fat
150 g/5 oz wholemeal flour
2 tbsp cold water
1 tbsp polyunsaturated oil

Filling
1 onion, finely chopped
25 g/¾ oz polyunsaturated margarine
100 g/3½ oz cooked red kidney beans
½ green pepper, sliced
1 egg
125 ml/4 fl oz semi-skimmed milk
100 g/3½ oz Cheddar cheese, grated
seasoning

Rub the fats into the flour, then add the water and oil, mixing to a dough with a round-ended knife. Leave the dough to rest for 10 minutes.

Preheat the oven to 180°C/350°F/gas 4.

Melt the margarine and fry the onion gently without browning for 5 minutes.

Roll out the pastry and line an 18 cm/7 in flan ring. Spread the onion over the pastry and arrange the beans and sliced pepper on top. Whisk together the egg, milk and cheese, and season. Pour over the flan case and bake for 35–40 minutes until set. Serve hot or cold. The flan can be frozen.

Chicken picnic flan

Serves 4

Each serving: 410 kcal/1715 kJ, 30 g (3 exchanges) carbohydrate, 4 g fibre, 21 g protein, 24 g fat

Pastry
40 g/1¹/₃ oz polyunsaturated
  margarine
35 g/1¹/₄ oz white vegetable fat
150 g/5 oz wholemeal flour
2 tbsp cold water
1 tbsp polyunsaturated oil

Filling
1 rasher lean bacon, finely chopped
1 small onion, finely chopped
150 g/5 oz cooked chicken meat
  (without skin) cut in chunks
1 egg
150 ml/5 fl oz semi-skimmed milk
3 tbsp skimmed milk soft cheese
¹/₂ tsp dried tarragon
seasoning

Rub the fats into the flour, then add the water and oil, mixing to a dough with a round-ended knife. Leave the dough to rest for 10 minutes.

Fry the bacon in its own fat until crisp, drain off any excess fat before adding the onion and cooking gently for a further 2–3 minutes.

Preheat the oven to 180°C/350°F/gas 4. Roll out the pastry and line an 18 cm/7 in flan ring. Spread the onion and bacon over the pastry and arrange the chicken pieces on top. Whisk together the egg, milk, cheese, tarragon and seasoning. Pour the mixture over the chicken and bake for 35–40 minutes until set. Serve hot or cold. The flan can be frozen.

Yoghurt drumsticks

Serves 4

Each serving: 100 kcal/420 kJ, negligible carbohydrate, negligible fibre, 15 g protein, 4 g fat

4 tbsp natural yoghurt
¹/₂ tsp paprika
¹/₂ tsp ground coriander

1 tsp tomato purée
seasoning
4 chicken drumsticks (without skin)

Stir the yoghurt, spices, tomato purée and seasoning until blended. Spoon this mixture over the chicken drumsticks, turning them over until well coated. Let the drumsticks marinate for 1–2 hours.

Preheat the oven to 160°C/325°F/gas 3 and cook the drumsticks for 30–40 minutes or until they are cooked through. Serve hot or cold.

Opposite: Yoghurt drumsticks (*top and in lunch box*); Pear and almond flapjacks (*left*, see page 99); Sandwiches (*right*): Carrot and cheese filling (see page 76), Liver sausage and pickle filling (see page 77), Cottage cheese and apricot filling (see page 77)

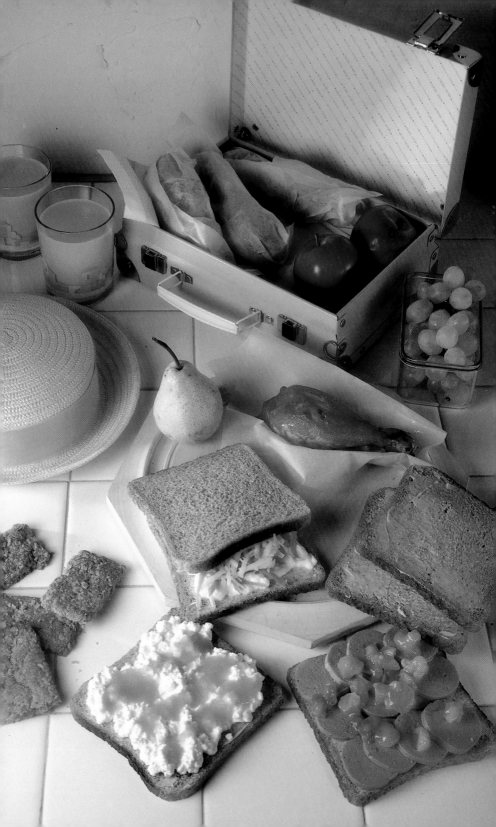

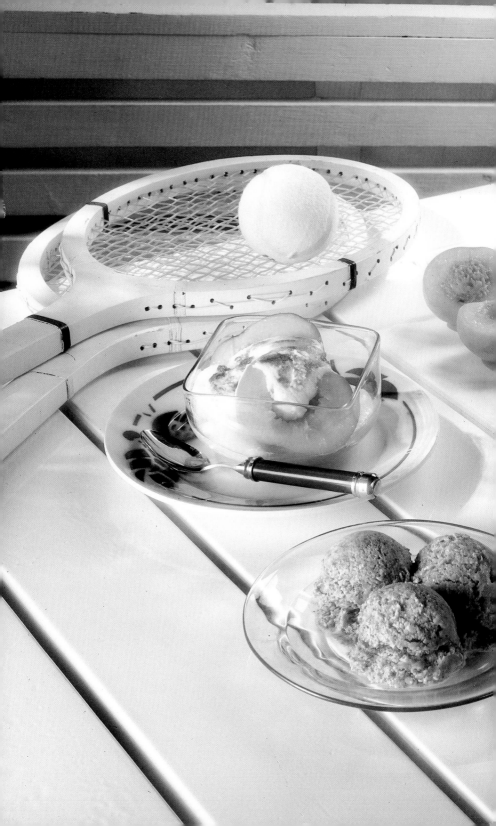

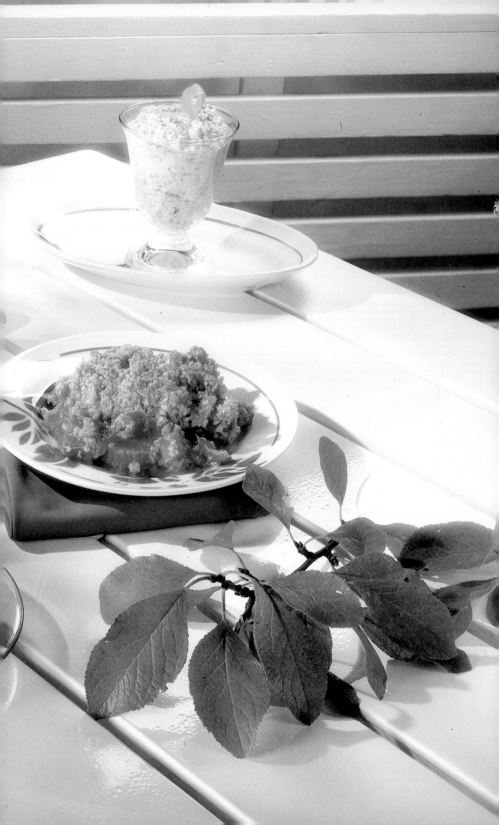

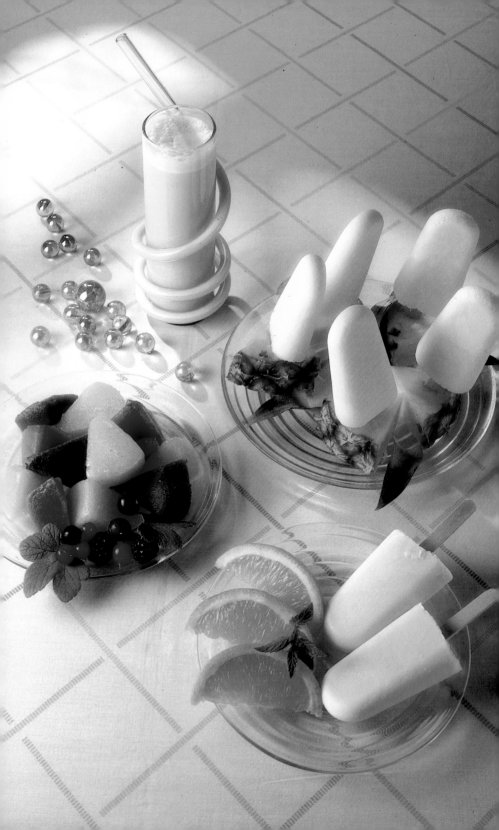

DESSERTS

Peach brûlée See photograph, page 82

Serves 6
Each serving: 90 kcal/380 kJ, 20 g (2 exchanges) carbohydrate, 2 g fibre, 4 g protein, negligible fat

6 ripe peaches, halved and stoned
300 ml/1/2 pint natural yoghurt
sugar-free sweetener equivalent
*   to 60 g/4 tbsp sugar*

15 g/1/2 oz castor sugar

Place the peaches cut-side down in a flat oven-proof dish. Mix the yoghurt and sweetener. Pour this over the peaches and sprinkle the fructose evenly over the top. Preheat the grill and place the dish under it until the fructose browns and caramelizes. Serve immediately.

Rhubarb, date and orange crumble See photograph, page 82

Serves 6
Each serving: 220 kcal/940 kJ, 30 g (3 exchanges) carbohydrate, 5 g fibre, 4 g protein, 11 g fat

450 g/1 lb rhubarb, sliced
100 g/3 1/2 oz dates, finely chopped
grated rind and juice of 1 medium-
*   sized orange*

Topping
75 g/2 1/2 oz wholemeal flour
75 g/2 1/2 oz rolled oats
1/2 tsp mixed spice
75 g/2 1/2 oz polyunsaturated
*   margarine*
sugar-free sweetener to taste

Preheat the oven to 190°C/375°F/gas 5.
Place the rhubarb in an ovenproof pie dish with the dates. Add the rind and juice of the orange.
Mix together the flour, oats and spices in a bowl and combine these with the margarine, using a fork, until well mixed. Spread the topping over the fruit and press down lightly. Bake for 35–40 minutes.
Sprinkle with sugar-free sweetener to taste, if necessary, when the pudding is served.

Previous page: Nutty whip (*top*, see page 90); Peach brulée (*centre left*); Rhubarb, date and orange crumble (*centre right*); Chocolate chip ice cream (*bottom*, see page 88)
Opposite: Blackcurrant milk shake (*top*, see page 101); Frozen fruit purées (*centre left*, see page 100); Pineapple yoghurt lollies (*centre right*, see page 101); Orange yoghurt lollies (*bottom*, see page 101)

Brown rice pudding

Serves 6

Each serving: 210 kcal/880 kJ, 30 g (3 exchanges) carbohydrate, negligible fibre, 8 g protein, 4 g fat

750 ml/1¹/₄ pints semi-skimmed
  milk
225 g/8 oz short-grain brown rice

sugar-free sweetener equivalent
  to 60 g/4 tbsp sugar
¹/₂ tsp ground nutmeg
1 egg, beaten

Bring the milk to the boil in a heavy-based saucepan. Sprinkle in the rice and stir. Cover tightly and simmer gently for about 50 minutes or until the rice is tender. Allow it to cool a little. Stir in the sweetener, ground nutmeg and beaten egg. Pour into a baking dish.

Preheat the oven to 180°C/350°F/gas 4. Bake the rice pudding for 30 minutes. Serve hot or use to make Fruit condés (see below).

Strawberry condé

Serves 6

Each serving: 150 kcal/620 kJ, 20 g (2 exchanges) carbohydrate, 2 g fibre, 7 g protein, 3 g fat

¹/₂ quantity of cold Brown rice
  pudding (see above)
300 ml/¹/₂ pint natural yoghurt

sugar-free sweetener to taste
400 g/14 oz strawberries, reserving 6
  whole strawberries for decoration

Mix together the cold rice pudding and yoghurt and sweeten if necessary. Quarter the strawberries, and arrange in layers with the rice mixture. Decorate with the reserved strawberries.

Raspberry condé

Serves 6

Each serving: 150 kcal/620 kJ, 20 g (2 exchanges) carbohydrate, 5 g fibre, 7 g protein, 3 g fat

Follow the recipe for Strawberry condé but replace the strawberries with 400 g/14 oz raspberries.

Orange condé

Serves 6

Each serving: 150 kcal/620 kJ, 20 g (2 exchanges) carbohydrate, 1 g fibre, 7 g protein, 3 g fat

Follow the recipe for Strawberry condé but replace the strawberries with 300 g/10¹/₂ oz sliced orange flesh.

Secret fruit mousse

Serves 6
Each serving: 110 kcal/450 kJ, 20 g (2 exchanges) carbohydrate, 7 g fibre, 8 g protein, negligible fat

250 g/9 oz stoned dried prunes, soaked in cold water for 4–6 hours
1 tbsp lemon juice
250 g/9 oz skimmed milk soft cheese

sugar-free sweetener equivalent to 30 g/2 tbsp sugar
150 ml/¼ pint natural yoghurt
dried egg white equivalent to 1 egg white

Simmer the prunes in their soaking water for 15–20 minutes. Sieve or liquidize the fruit with a little of the cooking liquid. Add the lemon juice. Beat the cheese and sweetener into the purée, then stir in the yoghurt. Whisk the egg white to soft peaks and gently fold into the prune mixture. Transfer to individual serving dishes and chill.

Mandarin crunch pudding

Serves 6
Each serving: 170 kcal/700 kJ, 20 g (2 exchanges) carbohydrate, 3 g fibre, 5 g protein, 8 g fat

50 g/1½ oz polyunsaturated margarine
200 g/7 oz wholemeal breadcrumbs (stale)
powdered or granular sugar-free sweetener equivalent to 60 g/4 tbsp sugar

300 g/10½ oz canned unsweetened mandarin oranges, drained
250 ml/9 fl oz natural yoghurt
sugar-free sweetener to taste

Melt the margarine in a large frying pan and fry the breadcrumbs over a high heat until well browned and crispy, stirring continuously. Allow them to cool, then stir in the sweetener. Reserve six mandarin segments for decoration. Purée or liquidize the remainder and mix these with the yoghurt, sweetening if necessary. Just before serving, layer the breadcrumbs with the yoghurt mixture in a serving dish or individual dishes. Decorate with the reserved mandarin segments.

Raspberry sorbet

Serves 6
Each serving: 50 kcal/210 kJ, 10 g (1 exchange) carbohydrate, 5 g fibre, negligible protein, negligible fat

50 g/1½ oz castor sugar*
450 ml/¾ pint water
225 g/8 oz fresh or frozen raspberries

juice of ½ lemon
dried egg white equivalent to 1 egg white

Set the freezer or refrigerator freezing compartment to the coldest setting.
Dissolve the castor sugar in the water and bring to the boil. Simmer for 5 minutes, then leave the syrup to cool.

Purée the raspberries and mix with the syrup and lemon juice. Transfer to a flat metal container, eg, a baking tin. Place in the freezer. When the sorbet has begun to freeze, remove from the freezer, whisk it well to break up the ice. Return to the freezer and repeat this process several times until a 'slush' of small ice crystals forms. Whisk the egg white to soft peaks and carefully fold it into the raspberry 'slush'. Transfer the mixture to an airtight plastic container and freeze finally. Allow the sorbet to thaw at room temperature for 15–30 minutes before serving.

*If fructose is used instead of castor sugar, use 50 g/1½ oz. Each portion will then yield 5 g (0.5 exchange) carbohydrate.

Vanilla ice cream

Serves 6
Each serving: 130 kcal/530 kJ, 5 g (0.5 exchange) carbohydrate, negligible fibre, 6 g protein, 9 g fat

4 egg yolks
600 ml/1 pint whole milk
1 tsp vanilla essence

sugar-free sweetener equivalent
to 75 g/5 tbsp sugar

Set the freezer or refrigerator freezing compartment to its coldest setting.

Beat the egg yolks with a little of the milk until smooth, then add the remaining milk. Transfer the mixture to a double boiler. (Alternatively, stand a saucepan in a frying pan of gently simmering water.) Stir constantly until the mixture thickens and coats the back of a wooden spoon. Cool the custard before adding the sweetener. Pour the custard into a shallow metal container and put in the freezer. When it is beginning to form ice crystals around the edge, remove from the freezer, beat or whisk well and then return it to the freezer. Repeat this process four or five times, until a thick 'slush' of small ice crystals forms. Finally transfer to an airtight plastic container and freeze.

Allow the ice cream to defrost for 30–45 minutes at room temperature before serving. If an ice cream–making machine is available, you will get an even better result.

Chocolate chip ice cream See photograph, page 82

Serves 6
Each serving: 130 kcal/530 kJ, 5 g (0.5 exchange) carbohydrate, negligible fibre, 6 g protein, 9 g fat

4 egg yolks
600 ml/1 pint whole milk
1 tsp vanilla essence

sugar-free sweetener equivalent
to 75 g/5 tbsp sugar
25 g/3/4 oz diabetic plain
chocolate, finely grated .

Make the ice cream exactly as described for Vanilla ice cream (see above). Stir the diabetic chocolate into the ice cream before the freezing process is begun.

Banana ice cream

Serves 6
Each serving: 150 kcal/620 kJ, 10 g (1 exchange) carbohydrate, negligible fibre, 7 g protein, 9 g fat

4 egg yolks
600 ml/1 pint whole milk
sugar-free sweetener equivalent
*   to 75 g/5 tbsp sugar*

3 small bananas (skinned
*   weight 150 g/5 oz)*
juice of 1/2 lemon

Make the custard as described for Vanilla ice cream (see opposite), adding the sweetener after cooking. Mash the bananas with the lemon juice and stir this into the vanilla custard. Freeze the ice cream in stages as described.

Brown bread ice

Serves 6
Each serving: 110 kcal/462 kJ, 15 g (1.5 exchange) carbohydrate, 2 g fibre, 5 g protein, 4 g fat

76 g/2½ oz fresh wholemeal
*   breadcrumbs*
50 g/1½ oz ground hazelnuts
25 g/¾ oz castor sugar*

300 g/10½ oz natural yoghurt
sugar-free sweetener equivalent
*   to 30g/2 tbsp sugar*
dried egg white equivalent to 3 eggs

Preheat the oven to 200°C/400°F/gas 7 and set the freezer or freezing compartment of the refrigerator to its coldest setting.

Mix the breadcrumbs with the ground hazelnuts, and spread evenly on to a baking tray. Cook in the oven for 20 minutes, stirring occasionally. Then sprinkle the castor sugar over the crumbs and return to the oven for a further 20 minutes. The mixture should be crisp and dry at the end of the cooking time. Allow it to cool.

Sweeten the yoghurt with the sweetener. Whisk the egg whites until stiff. Fold the crumbs and egg whites into the yoghurt, transfer to an airtight plastic container and freeze immediately. Allow the ice to thaw for 30 minutes before serving.

*If fructose is used instead of castor sugar, use 25 g/¾ oz. Each portion will then yield 10g (1 exchange) carbohydrate.

Spiced cheesecake

Serves 6
Each serving: 260 kcal/1088 kJ, 20 g (2 exchanges) carbohydrate, 2 g fibre, 7 g protein, 18 g fat

40 g/1⅓ oz polyunsaturated
*   margarine*
35 g/1¼ oz white vegetable fat
150 g/5 oz wholemeal flour
pinch salt
2 tbsp water
1 tsp polyunsaturated oil

2 egg yolks
350 g/12 oz skimmed milk soft
*   cheese*
sugar-free sweetener equivalent
*   to 45 g/3 tbsp sugar*
1/2 tsp ground allspice
1/2 tsp cinnamon

Preheat the oven to 200°C/400°F/gas 6.

Rub the fats into the flour and salt until the mixture resembles fine breadcrumbs. Add the water and oil and mix to a dough with a round-ended knife. Allow the dough to rest for 10 minutes before rolling it out and lining an 18 cm/7 in flan ring. Bake the pastry case for 15 minutes.

Beat together the egg yolks, cheese, sweetener and spices. Pile this mixture into the pastry case and bake for a further 30–35 minutes until set. Cool then chill in the refrigerator. Served chilled.

Baked bananas

Serves 6
Each serving: 110 kcal/460 kJ, 10 g (1 exchange) carbohydrate, 5 g fibre, 2 g protein, 6 g fat

*25 g/³/₄ oz polyunsaturated
  margarine*
*6 medium-sized ripe bananas, halved
  lengthways*

*sugar-free sweetener equivalent
  to 30 g/2 tbsp sugar*
grated rind and juice of ¹/₂ lemon
25 g/³/₄ oz flaked almonds

Preheat the oven to 180°C/350°F/gas 4.

Spread the margarine over the base and sides of a shallow oven-proof dish. Arrange the bananas on the base of the dish. Mix the liquid sweetener with the lemon rind and juice, and sprinkle over the bananas. Scatter the flaked almonds on top and bake for 15–20 minutes.

Nutty whip See photograph, page 82

Serves 4
Each serving: 130 kcal/550 kJ, 10 g (1 exchange) carbohydrate, 1 g fibre, 7 g protein, 5 g fat

50 g/1¹/₂ oz medium oatmeal
50 g/1¹/₂ oz hazelnuts, chopped
*finely grated rind and juice of
  ¹/₂ lemon*

300 ml/10 fl oz natural yoghurt
*sugar-free sweetener equivalent
  to 30 g/2 tbsp sugar*
dried egg white equivalent to 1 egg white

Mix the oatmeal with the hazelnuts and 'dry-fry' them in a frying pan, stirring continuously until brown. Cool the mixture.

Mix the lemon rind and juice with the yoghurt and sweetener. Whisk the egg white until stiff and fold it into the yoghurt with the oatmeal mixture. Transfer to four individual serving dishes and chill.

Raspberry mousse

Serves 6
Each serving: 50 kcal/210 kJ, 5 g (0.5 exchange) carbohydrate, 5 g fibre, 7 g protein, negligible fat

400 g/4 oz fresh or frozen raspberries
3 tsp gelatine
6 tbsp water
*100 g/3¹/₂ oz skimmed milk
  soft cheese*

*sugar-free sweetener equivalent
  to 45 g/3 tbsp sugar*
*125 ml/4 fl oz small carton
  natural yoghurt*
dried egg white equivalent to 2 egg whites

Purée the raspberries, reserving a few for decoration. Put the gelatine and water in a small saucepan and leave for 3–4 minutes until the gelatine swells.

Beat the cheese with the sweetener, then add the raspberry purée and the yoghurt and mix well. Whisk the egg whites to a stiff foam. Heat the gelatine, gently swirling the pan, until it melts and dissolves. Then add to the raspberry mixture, stirring constantly to disperse the gelatine. Fold in the whisked egg whites. Transfer to a serving dish or individual dishes and chill. This mousse can be frozen successfully; allow about 12 hours to defrost.

Apricot mousse

Serves 8
Each serving: 60 kcal/250 kJ, 10 g (1 exchange) carbohydrate, 6 g fibre, 4 g protein, negligible fat

200 g/7 oz dried apricots,
  soaked overnight in 450 ml/
  ¾ pint cold water
15 g/½ oz gelatine

3 tbsp lemon juice
4 tbsp skimmed milk soft cheese
dried egg white equivalent to 2 egg whites

Simmer the apricots in the soaking water until very soft, then purée or liquidize them with the cooking liquid. Soak the gelatine in the lemon juice in a small saucepan. Leave it to stand for 3–4 minutes, then heat gently until the gelatine has dissolved. Mix the gelatine and the cheese into the warm apricot purée, stirring thoroughly. Whisk the egg whites until soft peaks form. Fold the whisked whites into the apricot purée. Divide the mixture between eight individual serving dishes. Chill.

Apple 'sludge'

Serves 4
Each serving: 40 kcal/150 kJ, 5 g (0.5 exchange) carbohydrate, negligible fibre, 3 g protein, negligible fat

½ tsp cinnamon
sugar-free sweetener to taste
10 tbsp unsweetened apple purée

150 ml/¼ pint natural yoghurt
dried egg white equivalent to 2 egg whites

Mix the cinnamon and sweetener into the apple purée. Add the yoghurt, stirring in thoroughly. Whisk the egg whites until stiff and fold into the apple mixture carefully. Transfer to a serving dish or individual bowls and serve as soon as possible.

CAKES AND COOKIES

Apple mince pies

Makes 24
Each pie: 70 kcal/280 kJ, 10 g (1 exchange) carbohydrate, negligible fibre, 1 g protein, 4 g fat

Wholemeal shortcrust pastry
(see page 54)

Filling
2 tbsp mincemeat
4 tbsp apple purée, unsweetened
2 tbsp semi-skimmed milk for glazing

Preheat the oven to 180°C/350°F/gas 4.

Roll out the pastry to 5 mm/¼ in thickness. Stamp out twenty-four 7.5 cm / 3 in diameter circles, and twenty-four 6 cm/2½ in diameter circles, re-rolling as necessary. Place the larger circles in patty tins. Mix together the mincemeat and apple purée and put a teaspoonful of the mixture into each patty tin. Dampen the edges of the smaller circles of pastry and use to cover the pies. Press down firmly and pierce the top of each pie with a fork. Brush each with a little milk and bake for 25–30 minutes. Cool on a wire rack.

These pies can be frozen in an airtight container.

Carrot cake

Makes 16 squares
Each square: 170 kcal/720 kJ, 10 g (1 exchange) carbohydrate, 2 g fibre, 4 g protein, 13 g fat

150 ml/¼ pint polyunsaturated oil
sugar-free sweetener equivalent
*   to 90 g/6 tbsp sugar*
225 g/8 oz wholemeal flour
1 tsp mixed spice
2 tsp baking powder
3 eggs, beaten

225 g/8 oz carrot, finely grated
75 g/2½ oz chopped walnuts

Topping
2 tbsp skimmed milk soft cheese
1 tbsp natural yoghurt
sugar-free sweetener to taste

Preheat the oven to 180°C/350°F/gas 4.

Mix together the oil and sweetener and add to the flour, spice and baking powder. Beat in the eggs and then fold in the carrot and walnuts. Transfer to a greased 20 cm/8 in square cake tin base lined with greaseproof paper. Bake for 1–1½ hours until firm. Cool on a wire rack.

When the cake is cool, beat together the soft cheese and yoghurt, adding sweetener to taste, and spread over the cake before cutting into sixteen squares.

Opposite: Carrot cake (*top*); Apple mince pies (*bottom*)

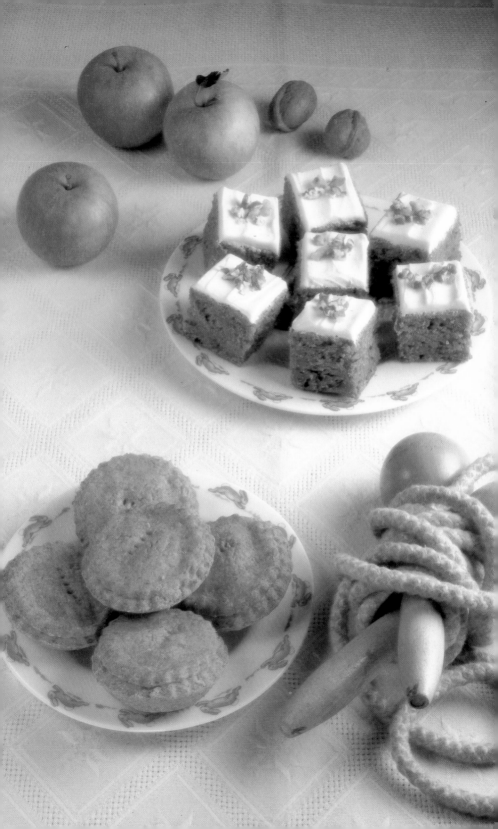

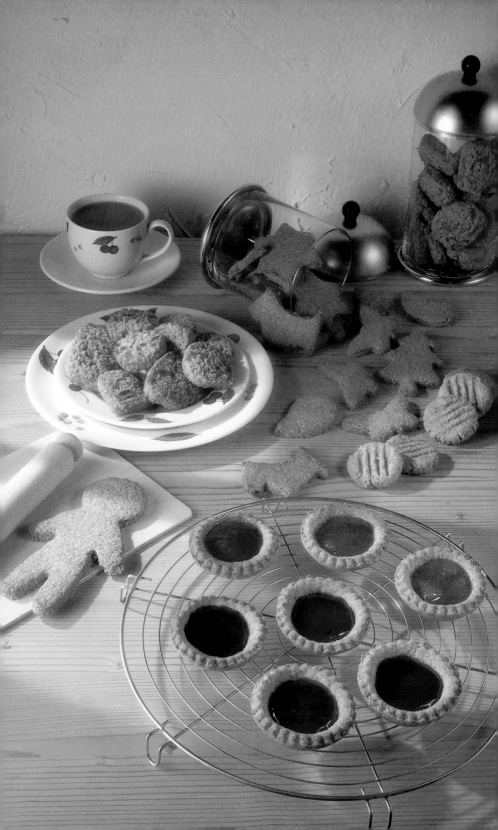

Cherry cookies

Makes 30
Each cookie: 65 kcal/273 kJ, 15 g (1.5 exchange) carbohydrate, negligible fibre, negligible protein, 3 g fat

100 g/3½ oz polyunsaturated
  margarine
100 g/3½ oz castor sugar*
½ tsp vanilla essence
50 g/1½ oz glacé cherries, chopped

100 g/3½ oz self-raising
  wholemeal flour
100 g/3½ oz rolled oats
2–3 tbsp semi-skimmed milk

Preheat the oven to 180°C/350°F/gas 4.

Cream together the margarine, castor sugar and vanilla essence until very light and fluffy. Add the cherries, flour and oats, and mix together. Add enough milk to form a soft dough. Knead lightly and shape into a sausage. Slice into thirty pieces and arrange widely spaced on a non-stick baking tray. Bake for 20–25 minutes. Cool on a wire rack.

*If using fructose instead of castor sugar, reduce the quantity to 75 g/2½ oz. Each biscuit will then yield 60 kcal/252 kJ, 10 g (1 exchange) carbohydrate.

Almond and orange biscuits

Makes 30
Each biscuit: 50 kcal/230 kJ, 5 g (0.5 exchange) carbohydrate, negligible fibre, 1 g protein, 4 g fat

100 g/3½ oz wholemeal flour
75 g/2½ oz medium oatmeal
50 g/1½ oz ground almonds

100 g/3½ oz polyunsaturated
  margarine
grated rind of 1 orange

Preheat the oven to 180°C/350°F/gas 4.

Put all the ingredients in a bowl and work with a fork until thoroughly blended. Then knead gently to a soft dough. Divide into thirty equal pieces; roll each into a ball and flatten on a non-stick baking tray. Bake for 10–15 minutes. Allow the biscuits to cool slightly before lifting on to a wire rack.

Rhubarb crumble cake

Makes 12 slices
Each slice: 160 kcal/672 kJ, 15 g (1.5 exchange) carbohydrate, 2 g fibre, 3 g protein, 10 g fat

200 g/7 oz rhubarb, cut into
  2.5 cm/1 in lengths
1 tbsp lemon juice
sugar-free sweetener equivalent to
  60 g/4 tbsp sugar

Base
100 g/3½ oz polyunsaturated
  margarine
75 g/2 oz castor sugar*
2 eggs, separated
1 tbsp water
100 g/3½ oz self-raising wholemeal flour

Opposite: Cherry cookies (*top left and in storage jar*); Almond and orange biscuits (*top right*); Jam tarts (*bottom*, see page 97)

Topping
25 g/³/₄ oz polyunsaturated margarine   1 tsp mixed spice
50 g/1¹/₂ oz coarse oatmeal

Preheat the oven to 180°C/350°F/gas 4.
Toss the rhubarb in the lemon juice and sweetener. Set aside.
Mix the topping ingredients with a fork until the margarine has blended.
Then make the base. Cream the margarine and castor sugar until light and fluffy.
Mix the egg yolks with the water and add gradually, beating well. Whisk the
egg whites to a foam and fold in with the flour. Transfer to a greased, sliding-
based 18 cm/7 in diameter cake tin. Put the rhubarb on top of the mixture and
sprinkle with the crumble topping. Stand on a baking tray and bake for 45–60
minutes. Leave to cool in the tin.

*If using fructose instead of castor sugar, reduce the quantity to 50 g/1¹/₂ oz. This
will yield 150 kcal/630 kJ, and 10 g (1 exchange) carbohydrate.

Cindy's coconut fruit squares

Makes 18
**Each square: 160 kcal/670 kJ, 10 g (1 exchange) carbohydrate, 1 g fibre,
4 g protein, 11 g fat**

8 tbsp polyunsaturated oil   50 g/1¹/₂ oz unsweetened shredded
2 eggs, beaten   coconut
1 tsp vanilla essence   25 g/³/₄ oz raisins
200 g/7 oz rolled oats   25 g/³/₄ oz wheatgerm
50 g/1¹/₂ oz sesame seeds   25 g/³/₄ oz unsalted peanuts, chopped

Preheat the oven to 180°C/350°F/gas 4. Oil a Swiss roll tin (25 x 28 cm/
10 x 11 in) lightly.
Whisk the oil, eggs and vanilla essence with a fork. Mix the remaining
ingredients in a bowl; pour in the oil mixture and beat well until thoroughly
mixed. Pour into the tin and bake for 20–25 minutes. Cool in the tin and cut
into eighteen squares.

Apple cake

Makes 12 slices
**Each slice: 110 kcal/450 kJ, 10 g (1 exchange) carbohydrate, 2 g fibre,
5 g protein, 5 g fat**

2 eggs, beaten   25 g/³/₄ oz skimmed milk powder
3 tbsp polyunsaturated oil   2 tsp baking powder
5 tbsp unsweetened, cooked apple   50 g/1¹/₂ oz sultanas
   purée   25 g/³/₄ oz wheatgerm
75 g/2¹/₂ oz wholemeal flour   1 tsp cinnamon
50 g/1¹/₂ oz soya flour

Preheat the oven to 180°C/350°F/gas 4.
Whisk the eggs and oil together and mix with the apple purée. Put all the
remaining ingredients into a bowl and mix thoroughly. Add the egg mixture and
blend together. Pour into a greased, 20 cm/8 in diameter cake tin, lined with
greaseproof paper, and bake for 1³/₄ hours until firm.

Choc-date cake

Makes 12 slices
**Each slice: 170 kcal/700 kJ, 20 g (2 exchanges) carbohydrate, 3 g fibre,
3 g protein, 9 g fat**

*100 g/3¹/₂ oz polyunsaturated
   margarine
150 g/5 oz stoned dates, finely
   chopped
150 ml/¹/₄ pint water*

*1¹/₂ tsp cocoa powder
1 egg, beaten
200 g/7 oz wholemeal flour
¹/₂ tsp ground cinnamon
1 tsp baking powder*

Preheat the oven to 190°C/375°F/gas 5.
   Put the margarine, dates, water and cocoa powder into a saucepan and heat slowly, stirring all the time until the margarine melts. Bring to the boil and simmer for 5 minutes. Allow the mixture to cool before adding the egg, flour, cinnamon and baking powder. Mix well and transfer to a greased 20 cm/8 in diameter cake tin. Bake for 1¹/₄ hours. Cool on a wire rack.

Jam tarts See photograph, page 94

Makes 30
**Each tart: 40 kcal/170 kJ, 5 g (0.5 exchange) carbohydrate, negligible fibre,
negligible protein, 2 g fat**

*Wholemeal shortcrust pastry
   (see page 54)*

*30 tsps (or 250 g/9 oz) sugar-
   free jam*

Preheat the oven to 180°C/350°F/gas 4.
   Roll out the pastry to 5 mm/ ¹/₄ in thickness. Stamp out thirty 7.5 cm/3 in diameter circles, re-rolling as necessary. Place the pastry circles in patty tins and put 1 tsp jam into each. Bake for 20–25 minutes. Cool on a wire rack.

Aduki bean brownies

Makes 20
**Each brownie: 50 kcal/220 kJ, 5 g (0.5 exchange) carbohydrate, 1 g fibre,
2 g protein, 3 g fat**

*50 g/1¹/₂ oz aduki beans, soaked
   in cold water overnight
450 ml/³/₄ pint water
1 tsp vanilla essence
1 tsp cinnamon
sugar-free sweetener equivalent to
   60 g/4 tbsp sugar*

*2 tbsp polyunsaturated oil
1 egg, beaten
100 g/3¹/₂ oz wholemeal flour
1 tsp baking powder
1 tbsp cocoa powder
40 g/1¹/₄ oz diabetic
   chocolate*

Preheat the oven to 180°C/350°F/gas 4.
   Drain the beans and place in a saucepan with the fresh water. Boil hard for 10 minutes then cover with a lid and simmer for about 1 hour until the beans are tender. Cool, then mash or liquidize the beans with the water, vanilla essence, cinnamon and liquid sweetener. Add the oil, egg, flour, baking powder and cocoa powder, and beat the mixture. Pour into a lightly oiled 20 cm/8 in square cake tin and cook for 45 minutes or until firm. Cut into twenty squares, allow to cool slightly, and lift them on to a wire rack.

Melt the chocolate on a plate in the oven for 2–3 minutes. Spread a little melted chocolate on to each square before they cool completely.

Apricot oatcake

Makes 24 squares
Each square: 120 kcal/490 kJ, 10 g (1 exchange) carbohydrate, 3 g fibre, 2 g protein, 7 g fat

150 g/5 oz dried apricots, soaked in
  300 ml/1/2 pint cold water overnight
1/2 tsp cinnamon
1 tbsp lemon juice

sugar-free sweetener to taste
175 g/6 oz polyunsaturated margarine
175 g/6 oz wholemeal flour
175 g/6 oz oatmeal

Simmer the apricots in the water with the cinnamon and lemon juice until soft. Purée the apricots and sweeten to taste.
   Preheat the oven to 190°C/375°F/gas 5.
   Melt the margarine and stir the flour and oatmeal into it. Spread half the mixture in a Swiss roll tin (25 x 28 cm/10 x 11 in), spread the apricot purée on top, cover with the remaining oat mixture and press down lightly. Bake for 30 minutes. Cut into twenty-four squares and allow to cool slightly before removing from the tin.

Banana and peanut oaties

Makes 16
Each oatie: 130 kcal/530 kJ, 10 g (1 exchange) carbohydrate, 2 g fibre, 3 g protein, 7 g fat

175 ml/6 fl oz unsweetened apple
  juice
25 g/3/4 oz raisins
25 g/3/4 oz dates, chopped
50 g/11/2 oz polyunsaturated margarine

1 medium-sized banana, mashed
6 tbsp crunchy peanut butter
200 g/7 oz jumbo oats

Preheat the oven to 180°C/350°F/gas 4.
   Bring the apple juice, raisins and dates to the boil in a small saucepan and simmer gently, stirring constantly, for 1–2 minutes until the mixture becomes thick and slightly sticky. Add the margarine to the pan and allow to melt over the heat. Mix in the mashed banana, peanut butter and finally the oats. Blend thoroughly before spreading the mixture evenly in a lightly oiled Swiss roll tin (25 x 28 cm/10 x 11 in) and pressing down lightly. Bake for 30 minutes or until firm to the touch.

Ginger nut cookies

Makes 35
Each cookie: 50 kcal/230 kJ, 5 g (0.5 exchange) carbohydrate, negligible fibre, negligible protein, 3 g fat

100 g/31/2 oz wholemeal flour
75 g/21/2 oz rolled oats
50 g/11/2 oz hazelnuts, ground
  or finely chopped

100 g/31/2 oz polyunsaturated
  margarine
25 g/3/4 oz castor sugar*
1 tsp ground ginger

Preheat the oven to 180°C/350°F/gas 4.

Put all the ingredients into a bowl and work with a fork until thoroughly blended. Then knead gently to a soft dough. Divide into thirty-five equal pieces; roll each into a ball and flatten with the hand on to a non-stick baking tray. Bake for 10–15 minutes. Allow to cool slightly before transferring to a wire rack.

*If fructose is used instead of castor sugar use 25 g/¾ oz but divide the mixture into 30 biscuits to give the equivalent exchanges as above.

Pear and almond flapjacks See photograph, page 81

Makes 15
Each flapjack: 120 kcal/504 kJ, 10 g (1 exchange) carbohydrate, negligible fibre, 1 g protein, 8 g fat

100 g/3½ oz rolled oats
50 g/1½ oz ground almonds
50 g/1½ oz dried pears, soaked in
cold water for 1 hour, drained
and chopped

100 g/3½ oz polyunsaturated
margarine
*50 g/1½ oz castor sugar**

Preheat the oven to 160°C/325°F/gas 3.

Mix the oats, ground almonds and dried pears together in a bowl. Melt the margarine and castor sugar in a saucepan, then pour over the oat mixture and mix well. Press the mixture into a lightly oiled Swiss roll tin (25 x 28 cm/10 x 11 in) and bake for 25–30 minutes, until golden. Cut into fifteen pieces but leave until completely cold before removing them from the tin.

*If fructose is used instead of castor sugar, use 50 g/1½ oz and cut the mixture into 20 pieces. Each flapjack will then yield 80 kcal/336 kJ and 5g (0.5 exchange) carbohydrate.

Plum slices

Makes 20
Each slice: 85 kcal/357 kJ, 10 g (1 exchange) carbohydrate, negligible fibre, 1 g protein, 8 g fat

100 g/3½ oz polyunsaturated
margarine
*100 g/3½ oz castor sugar**
2 eggs, separated
1 tbsp water

100 g/3½ oz self-raising wholemeal
flour
200 g/7 oz cooking plums, stoned
and halved

Preheat the oven to 180°C/350°F/gas 4.

Cream together the margarine and castor sugar until very light and fluffy. Mix the egg yolks with the water and add a little at a time to the creamed margarine, beating well after each addition. Whisk the egg whites to a foam and add to the batter, alternating with the flour, mixing and folding in gently. Spread the mixture into a Swiss roll tin (25 x 28 cm/10 x 11 in). Place the plums, cut side down, on top of the mixture. Bake for 30–35 minutes. Cool in the tin and cut into twenty slices.

*If fructose is used instead of castor sugar, reduce the quantity to 75 g/2½ oz and cut the cake into 10 slices. Each slice will then yield 80 kcal/336 kJ and 5 g (0.5 exchange) carbohydrate.

SHAKES AND LOLLIES

Blackcurrant purée See photograph, page 84

Makes 300 ml/¹/₂ pint
Total recipe: 140 kcal/590 kJ, 30 g (3 exchanges) carbohydrate, 44 g fibre, 5 g protein, negligible fat

500 g/1¹/₄ lb blackcurrants   *2 tbsp water*

Put the blackcurrants and water into a heavy-based saucepan, cover with a lid and cook slowly for 5–10 minutes until the fruit softens and the juice runs. Strain through a sieve and press gently to extract all the juice and some of the fruit pulp. The purée can be frozen in ice-cube trays or bags, so that a little can be thawed at a time for flavouring milk shakes, jellies, yoghurt or ice cream. Try using other fruits, such as rhubarb and orange.

Chocolate ice shake

Serves 4
Each serving: 110 kcal/440 kJ, 10 g (1 exchange) carbohydrate, negligible fibre, 7 g protein, 5 g fat

2 tsp cocoa powder
3 tbsp boiling water

600 ml/1 pint chilled, semi-skimmed milk
4 tbsp Vanilla ice cream (see page 88)

Mix the cocoa powder and water together. Then whisk this with the milk and 1 tbsp of the ice cream. Divide the remaining ice cream between four glasses and pour the chocolate-flavoured milk on top.

Peppermint cooler

Serves 4
Each serving: 80 kcal/340 kJ, 10 g (1 exchange) carbohydrate, negligible fibre, 7 g protein, 3 g fat

600 ml/1 pint chilled, semi-skimmed milk
3 tbsp crushed ice
1 tsp peppermint essence
3 tbsp skimmed milk soft cheese

sugar-free sweetener to taste
few drops of green food colouring (optional)
fresh mint leaves (to garnish)

Mix all the ingredients together in a blender and serve garnished with fresh mint leaves.

Blackcurrant milk shake See photograph, page 84

Serves 1
**Total recipe: 110 kcal/470 kJ, 10 g (1 exchange) carbohydrate, 1 g fibre,
9 g protein, 4 g fat**

*1 tbsp Blackcurrant purée (see opposite) 1 tbsp skimmed milk soft cheese
200 ml/7 fl oz semi-skimmed milk   sugar-free sweetener to taste*

Mix all the ingredients together in a blender for a few seconds and serve.

Banana milk shake

Serves 2
**Each serving: 140 kcal/570 kJ, 20 g (2 exchanges) carbohydrate, 1 g fibre,
7 g protein, 4 g fat**

*1 small banana, sliced   400 ml/14 fl oz semi-skimmed milk
2 tbsp orange juice*

Mix all the ingredients together in a blender for 30 seconds and serve.

Apricot milk shake See photograph, page 49

Serves 1
**Total recipe: 110 kcal/470 kJ, 10 g (1 exchange) carbohydrate, 1 g fibre,
7 g protein, 4 g fat**

*4 tbsp apricot purée   sugar-free sweetener to taste
1 tbsp lemon juice   200 ml/7 fl oz semi-skimmed milk*

Mix all the ingredients together in a blender for a few seconds and serve.

Orange yoghurt lollies See photograph, page 84

Makes 8
**Each lollipop: 30 kcal/110 kJ, 5 g (0.5 exchange) carbohydrate, negligible
fibre, 2 g protein, negligible fat**

*160 ml/5 1/2 fl oz unsweetened   300 ml/1/2 pint natural yoghurt
  orange juice   sugar-free sweetener to taste*

Mix the orange juice and yoghurt, and sweeten to taste with sweetener. Divide
between eight lollipop moulds and freeze.

Pineapple yoghurt lollies See photograph, page 84

Makes 8
**Each lollipop: 30 kcal/110 kJ, 5 g (0.5 exchange) carbohydrate, negligible
fibre, 2 g protein, negligible fat**

*160 ml/5 1/2 fl oz unsweetened   300 ml/1/2 pint natural yoghurt
  pineapple juice   sugar-free sweetener to taste*

Mix the pineapple juice and yoghurt, and sweeten to taste with sweetener.
Divide between eight lollipop moulds and freeze.

KIDS' COOKING

Cheesy toasts See photograph, page 111

Makes 12

Each toast: 100 kcal/420 kJ, 10 g (1 exchange) carbohydrate, 2 g fibre, 5 g protein, 5 g fat

2 tbsp semi-skimmed milk
15 g/¹/₂ oz polyunsaturated margarine
¹/₂ tsp dry mustard
black pepper
1 tsp vinegar

100 g/3¹/₂ oz mature Cheddar
  cheese, grated
12 x 25 g/³/₄ oz slices wholemeal
  bread, cut from a French stick
2 tomatoes, sliced

Put the milk, margarine, mustard, pepper and vinegar in a saucepan and bring the mixture to the boil slowly. Add the cheese and beat well until it has melted. Toast the bread on one side, turn over and spread the cheese mixture on to the untoasted side. Top each with a slice of tomato and grill for 5 minutes. Serve immediately.

Herb scones See photograph, page 49

Makes 8

Each scone: 150 kcal/640 kJ, 20 g (2 exchanges) carbohydrate, 2 g fibre, 3 g protein, 8 g fat

100 g/3¹/₂ oz self-raising wholemeal
  flour
100 g/3¹/₂ oz self-raising white flour
black pepper
50 g/1¹/₂ oz polyunsaturated
  margarine

1–2 tbsp chopped mixed fresh
  herbs (or 1–2 tsp dried)
120 ml/4 fl oz semi-skimmed milk
1 tbsp polyunsaturated oil

Preheat the oven to 220°C/425°F/gas 7.
   Mix the two flours and pepper in a bowl. Rub in the margarine with the fingertips until the mixture resembles fine breadcrumbs. Mix in the herbs. Add the milk and oil, and mix with a round-ended knife to a firm dough. Shape into a ball, kneading very lightly. Then flatten into a circle about 15 cm/6 in diameter, 2.5 cm/1 in thick. Score halfway through the dough to mark eight scones. Put on a floured baking tray and bake for 20 minutes until golden and firm. Cool on a wire rack.

Pizza baps

Makes 8
Each bap: 100 kcal/420 kJ, 10 g (1 exchange) carbohydrate, 2 g fibre, 6 g protein, 4 g fat

225 g/8 oz canned tomatoes
1 tbsp tomato purée
1/2 tsp dried oregano
1/2 tsp dried thyme
seasoning

4 wholemeal baps
4 small rashers lean bacon
4 mushrooms, sliced
50 g/1 1/2 oz Cheddar cheese, grated

Drain the tomatoes (save the juice for using in a soup or stew) and rub them through a sieve. Mix the tomato purée, herbs and seasoning into the tomato pulp. Split the baps and spread each with the tomato mixture. Top with a rasher of bacon, a sliced mushroom and some grated cheese. Cook under a hot grill until the cheese melts and the bacon is cooked. Serve immediately.

Sandwich pie

Serves 4
Each serving: 240 kcal/1010 kJ, 20 g (2 exchanges) carbohydrate, 5 g fibre, 15 g protein, 10 g fat

3 tomatoes, sliced
6 slices wholemeal bread
75 g/2 1/2 oz Edam cheese, grated
1/2 tsp dried basil

2 eggs
300 ml/1/2 pint semi-skimmed milk
pepper
1 tsp French mustard

Preheat the oven to 180°C/350°F/gas 4.
Reserve six tomato slices. Make three rounds of sandwiches, using the grated cheese and remaining tomato and sprinkling the basil over the filling. Cut each sandwich into four triangles and arrange in overlapping rows in a shallow ovenproof dish. Whisk the eggs, milk, pepper and mustard together with a fork. Pour the mixture over the sandwiches. Garnish with the reserved tomato slices and bake for 45 minutes.

Hamburgers

Makes 6
Each burger: 210 kcal/900 kJ, 20 g (2 exchanges) carbohydrate, 4 g fibre, 21 g protein, 6 g fat

450 g/1 lb lean minced beef
1 egg, beaten

seasoning
6 x 25 g/3/4 oz wholemeal baps, split

Mix the beef, egg and seasoning together and divide into six equal portions. Mould each portion into a flat hamburger with wet hands. Grill the burgers for 7 minutes on each side and serve in the split baps.

Lamb kebabs

Makes 4

Each kebab: 140 kcal/600 kJ, 5 g (0.5 exchange) carbohydrate, 1 g fibre, 17 g protein, 7 g fat

300 g/10¹/2 oz lean lamb, cut into 16 even-sized pieces
2 small onions (or 8 button onions), quartered
2 tomatoes, quartered
1 green pepper, cut into 12 slices

4 tsp fresh chopped mint
1 tsp fresh rosemary
2 tbsp lemon juice
seasoning

Thread the lamb and vegetables alternately on to four skewers and sprinkle with the herbs, lemon juice and seasoning. Cook under a hot grill or over a barbecue for 15–20 minutes, turning regularly.

Chicken kebabs   See photograph, page 111

Makes 4

Each kebab: 100 kcal/420 kJ, negligible carbohydrate, 1 g fibre, 17 g protein, 3 g fat

300 g/10¹/2 oz chicken breast (without skin) cut into 16 even-sized pieces
1 red pepper, cut into 16 even-sized pieces
1 courgette, cut into 16 even-sized pieces

16 small button mushrooms or 8 halved
¹/2 tsp dried thyme
2 tbsp lemon juice
seasoning

Thread the chicken, pepper, courgette and mushrooms alternately on to four skewers. Sprinkle the thyme, lemon juice and seasoning over the kebabs. Cook under a hot grill or over a barbecue for 15–20 minutes, turning regularly.

Bacon rolls

Makes 30

Each roll: 80 kcal/320 kJ, negligible carbohydrate, negligible fibre, 3 g protein, 7 g fat

15 rashers lean streaky bacon, rinds removed
225 g/8 oz low-fat sausagemeat

1 small onion, grated
1 tsp dried mixed herbs
seasoning

Cut each bacon rasher in half and stretch a little, using the back of a knife. Mix the grated onion, herbs and seasoning thoroughly with the sausagemeat and divide it into thirty small portions. Roll each piece of sausagemeat up in a half-rasher of bacon and thread on to a skewer. Cook under a grill or over a barbecue for 10–15 minutes until cooked through. Serve hot.

Sloppy joes

Serves 4
Each serving: 260 kcal/1080 kJ, 30 g (3 exchanges) carbohydrate, 9 g fibre, 25 g protein, 6 g fat

350 g/12 oz minced lean beef
1 onion, finely chopped
1 tsp dried mixed herbs
150 ml/¼ pint water

225 g/8 oz canned baked beans
*   in tomato sauce*
4 wholemeal baps

Cook the mince in a frying pan, gently at first to release the fat. Drain off any excess, then turn up the heat to brown it well. Add the onion and cook more gently for 5 minutes to soften it. Add the herbs and water, cover the pan and simmer gently for 30 minutes. Stir occasionally and add a little water if the mixture becomes too dry. Add the beans and bring to the boil again. Split the baps and divide the bean and mince mixture between them. Messy but fun!

Sausage and vegetable casserole

Serves 4
Each serving: 280 kcal/1170 kJ, 30 g (3 exchanges) carbohydrate, 5 g fibre, 15 g protein, 12 g fat

1 tbsp polyunsaturated oil
1 medium-sized onion, chopped
2 leeks, chopped
2 carrots, diced
3 celery stalks, diced
400 g/14 oz canned tomatoes,
*   chopped with juice*
300 ml/½ pint stock

1 tsp dried mixed herbs
225 g/8 oz low-fat pork sausages, cut
*   into 2.5 cm/1 in thick slices*
seasoning
2 medium-sized potatoes,
*   unpeeled, washed and diced*
50 g/1½ oz Edam cheese, grated

Heat the oil in a flameproof casserole or saucepan. Add the onion, leeks, carrots and celery. Cover with a lid and cook slowly for 10 minutes, stirring occasionally. Add the tomatoes, stock and herbs and bring to the boil. Add the sausages to the pan. Season and simmer for 30 minutes. Add the potatoes and cook for a further 30 minutes until they are tender. Serve with grated cheese sprinkled over the top.

Easy fruit cake

Makes 14 slices
Each slice: 140 kcal/580 kJ, 20 g (2 exchanges) carbohydrate, 2 g fibre, 3 g protein, 7 g fat

100 g/3½ oz polyunsaturated
*   margarine*
200 g/7 oz dried mixed fruit
150 ml/¼ pint water

1 egg, beaten
200 g/7 oz wholemeal flour
1 tsp mixed spice
1 tsp baking powder

Preheat the oven to 190°C/375°F/gas 5.

Put the margarine, dried fruit and water in a saucepan and heat gently until the fat has melted. Bring to the boil and simmer for 5 minutes. Allow to cool. Stir in the beaten egg, followed by the flour, spices and baking powder. Mix thoroughly and transfer to a greased 20 cm/8 in diameter cake tin base lined with greaseproof paper. Bake for 1¼ hours or until firm. Allow to cool a little before turning out.

Chocolate crunchies

Makes 16

Each crunchy: 50 kcal/220 kJ, 10 g (1 exchange) carbohydrate, negligible fibre, negligible protein, 3 g fat

50 g/1½ oz polyunsaturated margarine

50 g/1½ oz diabetic chocolate
100 g/3½ oz toasted wheatflakes

Melt the margarine and chocolate in a saucepan over a low heat. Stir to mix them together before adding the wheatflakes. Keep stirring until the flakes are coated. Divide the mixture between sixteen paper cake cases. Chill in the refrigerator before serving.

Lemon ice See photograph, page 111

Serves 4

Each serving: 50 kcal/220 kJ, 5 g (0.5 exchange) carbohydrate, negligible fibre, 7 g protein, negligible fat

grated rind and juice of 1 lemon
300 ml/½ pint natural yoghurt
3 tbsp skimmed milk soft cheese

sugar-free sweetener equivalent to 60 g/4 tbsp sugar
2 egg whites

Set the freezer or freezing compartment of the refrigerator to maximum.

Mix together the lemon rind and juice, yoghurt, cheese and sweetener. Whisk the egg whites until stiff and fold carefully into the yoghurt mixture. Turn into an airtight container and freeze.

Allow to defrost at room temperature for 30 minutes before serving.

PARTY COOKING

Birthday cakes

Most children like to have a special cake to celebrate their birthday and this is often the central feature of the party table. The foundation of such a cake is usually a basic sponge of some kind. The recipe below contains no sugar at all, the one on page 108 substitutes fructose. Remember when making a party cake that the children will be unlikely to eat very large slices so do not make too much.

Cakes can be decorated in numerous ways. Almond paste may be used to cover the cake as well as to mould into various decorative shapes. It can easily be coloured by kneading in edible food colourings (available in paste or liquid form) to give a bright appearance. See page 108 for the recipe for reduced-sugar Almond paste.

If a soft icing is preferred, the Soft cheese icing (see page 108) can also be coloured and used as a filling or a topping, but it is not really suitable for piping. A fruitier filling can be made by adding apricot purée to the basic recipe. The Chocolate cheese topping (see page 115) is another alternative.

There are vast numbers of non-edible items which can successfully be used to decorate birthday cakes: candle holders, ribbons, paper or plastic flowers, or even small toys such as figures or cars.

Sugarless sponge cake

Makes 10 slices
Each slice: 120 kcal/512 kJ, 10 g (1 exchange) carbohydrate, negligible fibre, 2 g protein, 10 g fat

100 g/3¹/2 oz polyunsaturated
margarine, melted
sugar-free sweetener equivalent to
60 g/4 tbsp sugar
5 drops vanilla essence

2 eggs, separated
1 tbsp water
100 g/3¹/2 oz self-raising wholemeal
flour

Preheat the oven to 190°C/375°F/gas 5. Lightly oil and line with greaseproof paper two 15 cm/6 in diameter sandwich tins.

Melt the margarine and allow it to cool before adding the sweetener, vanilla essence, egg yolks and water. Whisk up the mixture with a fork to blend thoroughly. Whisk the egg whites until they form soft peaks. Stir the flour into the margarine mixture, blending well. Then fold in the egg whites quickly, taking care not to beat or stir too hard at this stage. Divide the mixture between the two tins and bake for 15–20 minutes until firm. Cool on a wire rack.

Basic wholemeal sponge cake

Makes 12 slices

Each slice: 140 kcal/588 kJ, 15 g (1.5 exchange) carbohydrate, negligible fibre, 2 g protein, 8 g fat

*100 g/3½ oz polyunsaturated
  margarine*
100g /3½ oz castor sugar*

2 eggs, separated
1 tbsp water
100 g/3½ oz wholemeal flour

Preheat the oven to 180°C/350°F/gas 4. Lightly oil and line with greaseproof paper the bases of two 15 cm/6 in diameter sandwich tins.

Cream the margarine and the castor sugar until very light and fluffy. Mix the egg yolks with the water and add gradually to the creamed mixture, beating well after each addition. Whisk the egg whites until they form soft peaks and add these with the flour, mixing and folding in very gently. Divide the mixture between the prepared sandwich tins and bake until firm and golden — about 35–40 minutes. Transfer the cooked cakes to a wire cooling rack. When they are cool, fill, ice and decorate as required.

This mixture can also be baked in cake tins of other shapes with similar capacity.

*If fructose is used instead of castor sugar, reduce the quantity to 75 g/2½ oz and cut the cake into 10 slices. Each slice will then yield 152 kcal/632 kJ and 10g (1 exchange) carbohydrate.

Soft cheese icing

Covers and fills 10 slices

Each slice: 8 kcal/37 kJ, negligible carbohydrate, negligible fibre, 2 g protein, negligible fat

*100 g/3½ oz skimmed milk soft
  cheese*
2 tbsp natural yoghurt

*sugar-free sweetener equivalent to
  1 tbsp sugar*

Stir all the ingredients together until blended.

Do not 'ice' the cake too far in advance as the icing will dry out and become cracked.

Dippers See photograph, page 112

Any of the following vegetables can be used for dipping in the savoury dips below. Cut them into smallish pieces – large enough for just one mouthful.

The carbohydrate values of all these are considered to be negligible.

cabbage strips	courgette	Iceberg lettuce
carrots	cucumber	mushrooms
cauliflower	fennel	radish
celery	green pepper	red pepper

Fruit, crisps and biscuits are also suitable, but these provide more carbohydrate and so would need to be taken into account when working out carbohydrate exchanges. Choose wholemeal crisps, crackers and biscuits, and leave the skin on fruit wherever possible.

Split pea dip

Serves 4
Each serving: 190 kcal/790 kJ, 20 g (2 exchanges) carbohydrate, 4 g fibre, 9 g protein, 8 g fat

150 g/5 oz yellow split peas
300 ml/¹/₂ pint water
2 tbsp polyunsaturated oil

juice of ¹/₂ lemon
2 tbsp natural yoghurt
seasoning

Put the peas and water into a saucepan and bring to the boil. Simmer gently, uncovered, for about 40 minutes or until the peas are very tender. Drain away any excess water and then mash the peas with a potato masher. Mix in all the other ingredients and season to taste. Serve with a selection of 'dippers' (see above).

Cottage cheese and pineapple dip

Serves 4
Each serving: 40 kcal/170 kJ, 5 g (0.5 exchange) carbohydrate, negligible fibre, 5 g protein, negligible fat

100 g/3¹/₂ oz fresh or unsweetened
canned pineapple

8 tbsp skimmed milk soft cheese
4 tbsp natural yoghurt

Chop the pineapple very finely and mix with the cheese and yoghurt. Serve with a selection of 'dippers' (see above).

Smoked mackerel dip

Serves 6
Each serving: 150 kcal/650 kJ, negligible carbohydrate, negligible fibre, 15 g protein, 10 g fat

Follow the recipe for Smoked mackerel pâté (see page 77) but add an extra 2 tbsp natural yoghurt. Extra seasoning may be necessary too. Serve with a selection of 'dippers' (see above).

Tuna dip   See photograph, page 112

Serves 4

Each serving: 80 kcal/320 kJ, negligible carbohydrate, negligible fibre, 17 g protein, negligible fat

200 g/7 oz canned tuna fish in brine,
*   drained*
6 tbsp skimmed milk soft cheese
2 tbsp natural yoghurt

1 tsp soy sauce
1 tsp horseradish sauce
seasoning

Mash up the tuna with a fork. Blend the fish with all the other ingredients until smooth and creamy. This can be done more quickly in a food processor or liquidizer but it is possible to do so by hand, beating well with a wooden spoon. Serve with a selection of 'dippers' (see page 109).

Cheese and pickle dip

Serves 2

Each serving: 130 kcal/540 kJ, 5 g (0.5 exchange) carbohydrate, negligible fibre, 10 g protein, 9 g fat

4 tbsp semi-skimmed milk
50 g/1¹/₂ oz Cheddar cheese, grated

2 tbsp skimmed milk soft cheese
1 tbsp pickle

Bring the milk to the boil in a saucepan, then remove it from the heat and add the cheeses and the pickle. Beat well and return to the heat, stirring constantly until the cheeses have melted. Leave to cool before serving with a selection of 'dippers' (see page 109).

Houmous

Serves 4

Each serving: 230 kcal/990 kJ, 20 g (2 exchanges) carbohydrate, 6 g fibre, 10 g protein, 12 g fat

425 g/15 oz canned chick peas
juice of 1 lemon
3 tbsp tahini paste

1 clove garlic, crushed
2 tbsp polyunsaturated oil
seasoning

Drain the chick peas but reserve the juice. Blend or liquidize all the ingredients together to form a smooth paste. Add enough of the reserved juice to give a consistency suitable for 'dipping'. Houmous freezes well. Serve with a selection of 'dippers' (see page 109).

Opposite: Chicken kebabs (*top left*, see page 104); Lemon ice (*top right*, see page 106); Cheesy toasts (*bottom*, see page 102)

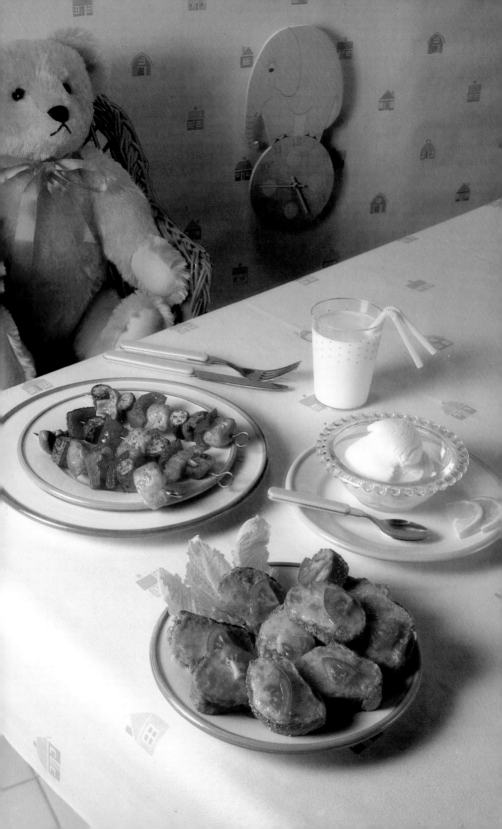

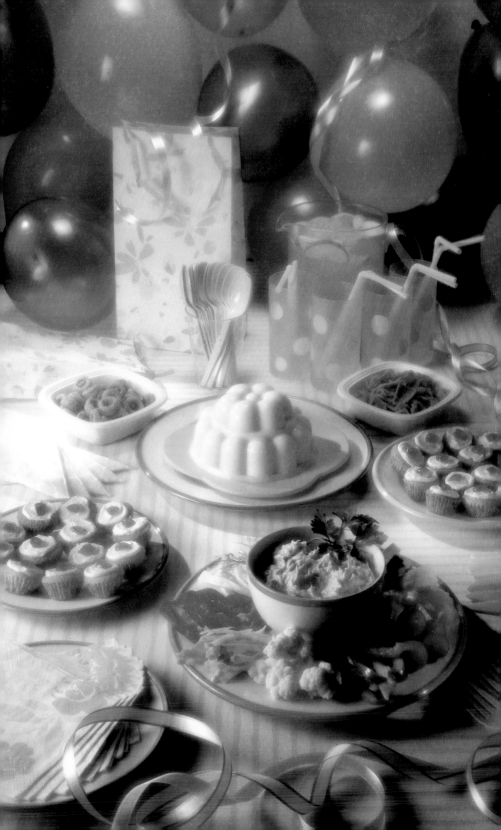

Cheesy nibbles

Makes 40 biscuits
Each biscuit: 30 kcal/110 kJ, 5 g (0.5 exchange) carbohydrate, negligible fibre, negligible protein, 2 g fat

50 g/1¹/2 oz polyunsaturated margarine
100 g/3¹/2 oz wholemeal flour
seasoning
¹/2 tsp dry mustard

50 g/1¹/2 oz Cheddar cheese, grated
1 egg yolk
1–2 tsp water

Preheat the oven to 180°C/350°F/gas 4.

Work the margarine into the flour, using a fork, until well mixed. Add the seasonings and cheese, and mix well. Add the egg yolk and water, and stir with a round-ended knife. Knead the mixture to form a stiff dough. Chill in the refrigerator for 10–15 minutes.

Roll out the dough on a floured surface to 5 mm/¹/4 in thickness and cut into forty fancy shapes or 3.5 cm/1¹/2 in diameter biscuits, re-rolling as necessary. Place these on a baking tray and bake for 10–15 minutes until crisp. Cool on a wire rack and store in an airtight container.

Split pea 'nuts'

Total recipe: 310 kcal/1300 kJ, 60 g (6 exchanges) carbohydrate, 12 g fibre, 22 g protein, 1 g fat

100 g/3¹/2 oz yellow split peas,
  soaked in cold water overnight

paprika
1 tsp lemon juice

Drain the split peas thoroughly, then dry them in a tea towel. Spread on a baking tray and cook in the oven 180°C/350°F/gas 4 for about 30 minutes until the peas are crispy. Sprinkle with paprika and the lemon juice. Cool and serve as 'nibbles'.

Pineapple yoghurt jelly

Serves 4
Each serving: 110 kcal/480 kJ, 20 g (2 exchanges) carbohydrate, negligible fibre, 9 g protein, negligible fat

400 ml/14 fl oz unsweetened
  pineapple juice
25 g/³/4 oz gelatine

300 ml/¹/2 pint natural yoghurt
sugar-free sweetener to taste

Put half the pineapple juice into a small saucepan, sprinkle in the gelatine and leave it to stand for 4 minutes. Heat gently, swirling the pan until the gelatine dissolves. Remove from the heat. Pour in the remaining juice and the yoghurt, and sweeten if necessary, stirring well. Pour into a 600 ml/1 pint jelly mould or a serving dish and chill in the refrigerator until set.

Opposite: Party fruit fizz (*top*, see page 115); Pineapple yoghurt jelly (*centre*); Party fairy cakes (*centre left and right*, see page 114); Tuna dip and dippers (*bottom*, see page 110 and 109)

Party fairy cakes See photograph, page 112

Makes 40
Each cake: 40 kcal/170 kJ, 5 g (0.5 exchange) carbohydrate, negligible fibre, negligible protein, 2 g fat

40 petits fours paper cake cases
100 g/3½ oz polyunsaturated margarine
100 g/3½ oz castor sugar*
2 eggs, separated
1 tbsp water
100 g/3½ oz self-raising wholemeal flour

Topping
50 g/1½ oz skimmed milk soft cheese
sugar-free sweetener equivalent to 15 g/1 tbsp sugar
few drops of food colouring (optional)
10 glacé cherries, quartered

Preheat the oven to 160°C/325°F/gas 3. Arrange the petits fours cases on baking trays.

Cream the margarine and castor sugar together until very light and fluffy. Beat in the egg yolks and water. Whisk the egg whites until stiff and fold them into the mixture gently with the flour. Mix gently but thoroughly until all the ingredients are combined. Place teaspoonfuls of the mixture into the paper cases and bake for 15 minutes. Cool on a wire rack.

Add the sweetener and colouring (if used) to the cheese and spread a little on top of the cooled cakes. Decorate the top of each cake with a quarter of a cherry.

*If fructose is used instead of castor sugar, reduce the quantity to 75 g/2½ oz. This will produce only a negligible decrease in the carbohydrate value.

Red grape jelly

Serves 10
Each serving: 60 kcal/270 kJ, 10 g (1 exchange) carbohydrate, negligible fibre, 2 g protein, negligible fat

1 litre/1¾ pint carton red grape juice
30 g/1 oz gelatine

sugar-free sweetener to taste (optional)

Put 150 ml/¼ pint of the juice into a small saucepan and sprinkle in the gelatine. Leave it to soak for 4 minutes, then heat gently, swirling the pan until the gelatine dissolves. Add the remaining juice, stirring, and sweeten to taste. Stir very thoroughly and then transfer to a mould or ten individual dishes. Chill in the refrigerator to set.

Chocolate orange crumb cake

Makes 12 squares
Each square: 150 kcal/640 kJ, 10 g (1 exchange) carbohydrate, 1 g fibre, 2 g protein, 12 g fat

200 g/7 oz unsweetened wholemeal bran biscuits
125 g/4½ oz polyunsaturated margarine

½ tsp cocoa powder
sugar-free sweetener equivalent to 2 tbsp/30 g sugar
grated rind of 1 orange

Crush the biscuits finely by placing them in a plastic bag and running a rolling pin over them.

Melt the margarine with the remaining ingredients. Add the crumbs to the melted margarine and mix thoroughly. Press the mixture into an 18 cm/7 in square cake tin and chill until very firm. Cut into twelve squares.

Chocolate cake with chocolate cheese topping

Makes 16 squares
Each square: 120 kcal/504 kJ, 5 g (0.5 exchange) carbohydrate, negligible fibre, 3 g protein, 7 g fat

100 g/3½ oz polyunsaturated
   margarine
100g /3½ oz castor sugar*
2 eggs, separated
1 tbsp cocoa powder
1 tbsp boiling water
100 g/3½ oz self-raising wholemeal
   flour

Topping
50 g/1½ oz plain diabetic chocolate,
   broken into small pieces
3 tbsp skimmed milk soft cheese
sugar-free sweetener equivalent
   to 15 g/1 tbsp sugar

Lightly oil and line with greaseproof paper the base of an 18 cm/7 in square cake tin. Preheat the oven to 190°C/375°F/gas 5.

Cream the margarine and castor sugar together until very light and fluffy. Beat in the egg yolks. Mix the cocoa powder with the boiling water and then beat this in too. Whisk the egg whites until stiff. Add the egg whites and flour to the mixture, folding in gently until they are thoroughly blended. Transfer to the cake tin and bake for 30–40 minutes until firm. Cool on a wire rack.

To make the topping, put the chocolate and cheese in a saucepan and heat gently, stirring all the time until the chocolate has melted. Add the sweetener. Then spread the topping over the cake. Cut into sixteen squares.

*If fructose is used instead of castor sugar, reduce the quantity to 75 g/2½ oz and cut the cake into 14 squares.

Frozen banana pops

Makes 6
Each 'pop': 40 kcal/180 kJ, 10 g (1 exchange) carbohydrate, 2 g fibre, 1 g protein, negligible fat

3 bananas
4 tbsp natural yoghurt
green food colouring

red food colouring
1 tsp chocolate sugar strands

Cut each banana in half and push a cocktail stick into each half. Freeze the bananas until firm.

Mix half the yoghurt with a few drops of green food colouring. Mix the remaining yoghurt with a few drops of red colouring. Take the bananas from the freezer and spoon over the coloured yoghurts to give a two-tone effect. The yoghurt will 'set' on to the cold banana. Sprinkle a few chocolate sugar strands over each and return to the freezer. Serve the banana pops frozen.

Party fruit fizz See photograph, page 112

Serves 6

Each serving: 40 kcal/180 kJ, 10 g (1 exchange) carbohydrate, negligible fibre, negligible protein, negligible fat

300 ml/1/2 pint unsweetened orange juice

250 ml/8 fl oz unsweetened apple juice
600 ml/1 pint chilled soda water

Mix the ingredients together and serve immediately.

Blackcurrant and mint fizz

Serves 6

Each serving: 5 kcal/20 kJ, negligible carbohydrate, 1 g fibre, negligible protein, negligible fat

6 tbsp Blackcurrant purée
(see page 100)
3 tbsp lemon juice
sugar-free sweetener to taste

1 litre/13/4 pints chilled sparkling mineral or soda water
fresh mint leaves

Mix all the ingredients together in a large jug. Sweeten to taste and float mint leaves on top. Serve immediately.

CARBOHYDRATE EXCHANGE LIST

Each of the foods listed below contains **10 g carbohydrate (1 exchange)**.

Foods are given in handy measures and weights. Measure the weight in grams where possible. The weights in ounces are given to the nearest equivalent. The tablespoon measurement is based on a level 15 ml spoon, the teaspoon on a level 5 ml spoon (such as the British Diabetic Association standard measuring spoons).

Foods marked with an * are high in fibre.

Food	Handy measure	Weight/volume
Bread		
Wholemeal bread*	1 thin slice from small loaf or 1/2 medium slice from large loaf (Note: 1 slice of most brands of pre-sliced large wholemeal loaves (eg, Windmill, Allinson) contain 15 g carbohydrate (1.5 exchanges))	25 g/3/4 oz
White bread	1 thin slice from small loaf	20 g/2/3 oz
Wholemeal roll or bap*	half a roll	25 g/3/4 oz
White or brown rolls	half a roll	20 g/2/3 oz
Biscuits		
Crispbread*	2 biscuits	15 g/1/2 oz
Digestive or wholemeal, large*	1 biscuit	15 g/1/2 oz
small*	2 biscuits	15 g/1/2 oz
Oatcake*	1 round oatcake	15 g/1/2 oz
Plain or semi-sweet (eg, Rich tea, Marie, Morning coffee)	2 biscuits	15 g/1/2 oz

Food	Handy measure	Weight/volume
Wholemeal crackers*(eg, Krackerwheat, Hovis, Farmhouse)	2 biscuits	15 g/¹/₂ oz
Cream crackers, water biscuits	2 biscuits	15 g/¹/₂ oz
Wholemeal shortbread*	1 finger	15 g/¹/₂ oz

Breakfast cereals

Allbran*	5 tbsp	20 g/²/₃ oz
Branflakes*	3 tbsp	15 g/¹/₂ oz
Cornflakes	5 tbsp	10 g/¹/₃ oz
Cubs*	14	15 g/¹/₂ oz
Muesli (unsweetened)*	2 tbsp	15 g/¹/₂ oz
Porridge oats (uncooked)*	3 tbsp	15 g/¹/₂ oz
Puffed wheat*	15 tbsp	15 g/¹/₂ oz
Rice Krispies	6 tbsp	10 g/¹/₃ oz
Shredded Wheat*	²/₃ biscuit	15 g/¹/₂ oz
Shreddies*	35	15 g/¹/₂ oz
Special K	8 tbsp	15 g/¹/₂ oz
Weetabix*	1 biscuit	20 g/²/₃ oz
Weetaflakes*	4 tbsp	15 g/¹/₂ oz

Other starchy foods

Chappati	1 small	25 g/³/₄ oz
Cornflour, custard powder, arrowroot	1 tbsp	10 g/¹/₃ oz
Pasta (macaroni etc) wholewheat* or white (dry) (boiled)	2 tbsp 4 tbsp	15 g/¹/₂ oz 40 g/1¹/₃ oz
Pitta bread (wholemeal*, white)	1 quarter	15 g/¹/₂ oz

Food	Handy measure	Weight/volume
Pudding rice, sago, tapioca, semolina (uncooked)	1 tbsp	10 g/$^1/_3$ oz
Rice, long-grained brown* or white (dry) (boiled)	1 tbsp 3 tbsp	10 g/$^1/_3$ oz 40 g/1$^1/_3$ oz
Shortcrust pastry wholemeal* or white	1 small square	20 g/$^2/_3$ oz
Spaghetti canned in tomato sauce	5 tbsp	80 g/2$^3/_4$ oz
Spaghetti (dry) wholemeal* white	20 short strands 6 long strands	15 g/$^1/_2$ oz 10 g/$^1/_3$ oz
Wholemeal flour*	2 tbsp	15 g/$^1/_2$ oz
White flour	1$^1/_2$ tbsp	10 g/$^1/_3$ oz

Milk and milk products

Dried skimmed milk	4 tbsp	20 g/$^2/_3$ oz
Evaporated milk (unsweetened)	6 tbsp	90 ml/3 fl oz
Semi-skimmed milk	1 glass	200 ml/7 fl oz
Skimmed milk	1 glass	200 ml/7 fl oz
Whole milk, fresh or long life	1 glass	200 ml/7 fl oz
Yoghurt, low fat natural	1 small carton	150 ml/$^1/_4$ pint

Vegetables (for other vegetables see table on page 22)

Beetroot, boiled*	4 medium slices	100 g/3$^1/_2$ oz
Parsnip*, boiled	1 medium	75 g/2$^1/_2$ oz
Peas, canned processed * (frozen - see Free food list)	7 tbsp	75 g/2$^1/_2$ oz
Plantains*, raw, peeled	1 small slice	35 g/1$^1/_4$ oz

Food	Handy measure	Weight/volume
Potato, boiled or jacket*	1 small (egg size)	50 g/1½ oz
mashed	1 small scoop	50 g/1½ oz
roast	1 small	40 g/1⅓ oz
chips	1 tbsp	25 g/¾ oz
Sweetcorn, canned, frozen*	5 tbsp	60 g/2 oz
Sweet potato*, raw	1 small slice	50 g/1½ oz
Yams, raw*	1 small slice	30 g/1 oz

Pulse vegetables*

Baked beans*	4 tbsp	75 g/2½ oz
Broad beans, boiled*	10 tbsp	150 g/5 oz
Dried beans*,		
raw	2 tbsp	20 g/⅔ oz
boiled	4 tbsp	60 g/2 oz
(eg haricot, soya, red kidney, butter, black-eyed)		
Lentils*,		
raw	2 tbsp	20 g/⅔ oz
cooked	4 tbsp	60 g/2 oz
Peas, chick peas*, dried,		
raw	2 tbsp	20 g/⅔ oz
boiled	5 tbsp	50 g/1½ oz

Fruit   (for other fruit, see table on page 22)

Fresh fruit weights are for the whole fruit, including skin, stone, core etc.
For fruit canned in water or natural juice, use figures for fresh fruit.

Apple*, dessert	1 medium	110 g/3¾ oz
Apple, cooking (stewed with sugar)	6 tbsp	125 g/4½ oz
Apricots*,		
fresh	3 medium	160 g/5⅔ oz
dried, raw	4 small	25 g/¾ oz
Banana*	1 small	90 g/3 oz
Cherries*	12	100 g/3½ oz

Food	Handy measure	Weight/volume
Dates*, dried, stoned	3	15 g/¹/₂ oz
Dried fruit* (sultanas, raisins, currants)	2 tbsp	15 g/¹/₂ oz
Figs*, dried	1	20 g/²/₃ oz
Grapes*	10 large	75 g/2¹/₂ oz
Mango*	¹/₃ large	100 g/3¹/₂ oz
Nectarine*	1 medium	90 g/3 oz
Orange*	1 large	150 g/5 oz
Peach*	1 large	125 g/4¹/₂ oz
Pear*	1 large	125 g/4¹/₂ oz
Pineapple*	2 rings	90 g/3 oz
Plums*, dessert cooking	2 large 4 medium	110 g/3³/₄ oz 180 g/6¹/₃ oz
Prunes*, stewed without sugar	4	50 g/1¹/₂ oz
Raspberries*	12 tbsp	175 g/6 oz
Strawberries*	15 medium	160 g/5²/₃ oz
Satsumas*	2 large	175 g/6 oz
Tangerines*	2 large	175 g/6 oz

Fruit juice

(Fruit juice should be taken as part of a meal, to delay absorption, rather than as a snack.)

Apple juice	6 tbsp	85 ml/3 fl oz
Grapefruit juice	8 tbsp	125 ml/4¹/₂ fl oz
Orange juice	7 tbsp	100 ml/3¹/₂ fl oz
Pineapple juice	6 tbsp (all roughly 1 small glass)	85 ml/3 fl oz

Food	Handy measure	Weight/volume
Snack foods		
(Note: many crisps and similar snacks contain 15 g carbohydrate (1.5 exchanges) for a small packet (about 25 g/³/₄ oz).		
Potato crisps	1 small yoghurt cartonful	15 g/¹/₂ oz
Savoury snacks (crisp-type, average)	1 small yoghurt cartonful	15 g/¹/₂ oz
Ice cream, plain	1 small brickette/scoop	50 g/1¹/₂ oz
Peanuts	1 medium packet	120 g/4¹/₃ oz
High-fibre crunchy bar ('muesli-type')	¹/₂ – ³/₄ bar	variable
Miscellaneous		
Beefburgers (no need to count small portion. 100 per cent meat burgers contain neg. carbohydrate)	2–4	185 g/6¹/₂ oz
Bournvita, Horlicks, Ovaltine	2 tsp	10 g/¹/₃ oz
Fish cakes	1	60 g/2 oz
Fish fingers	2	60 g/2 oz
Pork pie	1 thin slice	40 g/1¹/₃ oz
Sausage roll	1 small	30 g/1 oz
Sausages	1–2 thick, 3–4 thin	110 g/3³/₄ oz
Scotch egg	¹/₂	85 g/3 oz
Soup, thick or cream varieties	1 cup	200 ml/7 fl oz

ACKNOWLEDGMENTS

We should like to thank the following for their help and advice: Christine Clothier (Paediatric Dietitian), Sandra Lamont (Diabetic Dietitian), Kate Start (Honorary Secretary Paediatric Group of the British Dietetic Association), Penny Timbrell (Paediatric Dietitian), and the British Diabetic Association (10 Queen Anne Street, London W1M 0BD. Tel: 071 323 1531).

We are very grateful to Joan Soan and Heather Smith-Williams for typing the manuscript.

Rosemary Seddon and Jane Rossiter, 1987

The publishers would like to thank Ray Moller assisted by Sophie Butt for photography, Sue Russell for styling and Elaine Bastible for food preparation.

INDEX

Page numbers in *italic* refer to the illustrations